How Did We

Get So

FAT?

A guide
safely ob

Arnold

B

BL Publications, Detroit Lakes, MN 56501
218-846-2519/877-BOOKS11
www.blpbooks.com

Library of Congress Cataloging-in-Publication Data

Susser, Arnold J.
  How did we get so fat? : a guide for those who want to safely obtain their weight goals / Arnold J. Susser and Beth M. Ley.
       p. cm.
Includes bibliographical references and index.
  ISBN 0-9642703-0-7
  1. Weight loss. 2. Naturopathy. 3. Dietary supplements.
I. Ley, Beth M., 1964- II. Title.
  RM222.2 .S888 2001
  613.7--dc21

                                        2001000756

Printed in the United States of America

How Did We Get So Fat? is not intended as medical advice. Its intention is solely informational and educational. It is wise to consult a doctor before starting any weight loss program or for any illness or medical condition.

Credits:

Cover Design: Cuviello Graphic Design and
BL Publications

Proofreading and Editing: Renae Paulson and
Deborah Brenk

YOU NEED TO KNOW...
THE HEALTH MESSAGE

Do you not know that you are God's temple and that God's Spirit dwells in you? If anyone destroys God's temple, God will destroy him, For God's temple is holy and that temple you are.
1 Corinthians 3:16-17

So, whether you eat or drink, or whatever you do, do all to the glory of God.
1 Corinthians 10:31

Table of Contents

Introduction

Good health is the result of giving the body what it needs on a daily basis, while disease is the result of attempting to live without what the body needs. We are responsible for our own health, and should take control of it. If we are in control of our health, disease will not take control.

Our health depends on education.

Arnold J. Susser, R.P., Ph.D., has a nutrition counseling practice in Westfield, New Jersey, and for over 30 years has been involved with the nutritional aspects of health. He has seen first hand what proper nutritional support can do for his patients, for their health and numerous different health problems.

Dr. Susser is president of Great Life Labs, exclusive distributor of state of the art nutritional supplements, personally created by himself with his extensive background. He is a registered pharmacist, has a Ph.D. in nutrition and is a licensed naturopathic physician. In addition, Dr. Susser is the nutritional consultant for the trainers of the San Francisco Giants and the New York Yankees.

With a father and uncle as pharmacists, a career choice was simple for a young Arnold Susser. A graduate of Rutgers University, he was able to utilize his pharmacology and biochemistry background as he worked as a medical detail man for a large pharmaceutical company. He informed physicians as to the uses, side effects, etc. of new drugs to promote their sales for the company.

During this time he became very well acquainted with the problems, dangers, side effects, and complications of prescription drugs.

After 17 years in this position, Susser developed an ear infection which rapidly spread to the mastoid area behind the brain. Nervous about undergoing surgery, he looked into "alternative" approaches to improve his health. He incorporated the advice of his naturopathic physician (the occupation he would later enter) and altered his dietary intake, and gave up cigars and his pipe, coffee, refined sugar, etc. He began taking supplements to stimulate and support the immune system. After a few short weeks, the infection cleared. Much to the disbelief of many, he was able to avoid surgery completely.

This triggered a desire to pursue natural health and healing further. Until this time, he had assumed that what was taught in the medical and pharmacy schools was what health and medicine were all about. Susser feels that his serious illness which caused him to realize that there was more to health than drugs and surgery was no "chance" happening. He credits God for the events that led to his change of heart.

He returned to school and achieved his naturopathic degree and later his Ph.D. in nutrition. He then lectured at health symposiums, appeared on national radio and television shows, and was featured in numerous major newspapers on both the east and west coasts.

Eventually, this led to the start of his own nutrition practice in Westfield, New Jersey. After seeing the needs of his patients, and feeling unsatisfied with drugs, which have side effects, and also the available supplements on

6

the market at that time, he decided to formulate nutritional supplements that would give the body what it needs to produce its own chemicals, hormones, etc. for healing. These, in a sense, are the body's own "drugs," but without the dangers and side effects. For example, the body produces cortisone as a natural anti-inflammatory agent. It makes what it needs (providing it has the nutritional factors to make it from) and it doesn't over-produce. The body makes its own sleep chemicals, providing it has the nutrients to do so, and there is no risk of overdose. The body can even produce its own pain relievers, again, with the proper nutritional support. It produces interferon, known to fight all known viruses, and perhaps, even some unknown ones as well, through the immune system.

With nutritional support we can enhance our immune system, our ability to produce hormones (including the sex hormones) and all other healthy body chemicals.

Over the years, Dr. Susser has created more than 100 different nutritional formulations to enhance various systems of the body, for the use of his patients, and numerous individuals throughout the country and world. Through all this, Great Life Labs was created. Susser continues to act as chief executive officer and president, striving to produce the finest state-of-the-art products, using the highest quality ingredients possible.

"Among the many health problems that people have; cancer, headaches, allergies, arthritis, skin problems, etc, a concern which plagues almost every one of the patients I see, is a desire (and a need) to lose weight. When answering a questionnaire, 80% or more of my patients will check off

"lose weight" as one of their goals.

Obesity has reached epidemic status in our country. Weight problems threaten the lives of famous politicians, athletes, movie and television personalities and everyday people included.

The major reasons for weight problems are poor diet (malnutrition), overeating and lack of exercise. Over-processing of our foods and lack of nutrients in packaged foods also greatly contributes to our weight problems. Heredity also plays a role, but much can be done to aid and change the situation. Eating habits begin as a child. If your parents didn't teach you how to eat properly when you were young, those eating habits may carry through for the rest of your life. The same applies for your children.

A few simple weight-control rules:

1. Eat foods in their <u>NATURAL</u> state. Avoid processed, prepackaged, prepared foods. These are low in nutritional value, low in fiber and often high in sodium and fat.

2. Drink lots of water.

3. Eat less, don't stuff yourself. Eat small meals often, rather than a few large meals daily. Always eat a good breakfast. This increases your metabolic rate for the entire day.

4. Be active and/or get regular exercise.

HOW DID WE GET SO FAT?

According to the American Obesity Association, over 95 million Americans are above their ideal weight.

Obesity, defined as weighing over 20% of your ideal weight, is a major nutritional obstacle in America today. Leading medical authorities consider obesity to be the most widespread nutritional disorder in the United States. More than one-third of all adults and one in five children are obese. Today, 55% of adult Americans (97 million) are categorized as being over-weight or obese.

Each year, obesity causes at least 300,000 excess deaths in the U.S. and costs the country more than $100 billion. In spite of this, we are still fat. What is wrong with us?

Being obese and being overweight are not the same. A Body Mass Index (BMI) of 30 or greater is considered obese and a BMI between 25-29.9 is considered overweight. There are several variables that have an impact on a person's health risk relative to their BMI such as a person's waist size, whether a person smokes, the types of foods someone eats regularly, whether someone exercises regularly and the medical conditions associated with obesity including diabetes, high blood pressure, high cholesterol and coronary heart disease.

According to the American Obesity Association, obesity is an independent risk factor or an aggravating agent for more than 30 medical conditions including:

1. Osteoarthritis of knee & hip
2. Rheumatoid arthritis
3. Birth Defects
4. Breast Cancer in Women
5. Breast Cancer in Men
6. Cancers of the Esophagus & Gastric Cardia
7. Colorectal Cancer
8. Endometrial Cancer
9. Renal Cell Cancer
10. Cardiovascular Disease
11. Carpal Tunnel Syndrome
12. Chronic Venous Insufficiency
13. Daytime Sleepiness
14. Deep Vein Thrombosis
15. End Stage Renal Disease
16. Gallbladder Disease
17. Gout
18. Heat Disorders
19. Hypertension
20. Impaired Immune Response
21. Impaired Respiratory Function
22. Infections Following Wounds
23. Infertility
24. Liver Disease
25. Low Back Pain
26. Obstetric and Gynecological Complications
27. Pain
28. Sever Acute Biliary & Alcoholic Pancreatitis
29. Sleep Apnea
30. Stroke
31. Surgical Complications
32. Traumatic Injuries to Teeth
33. Type 2 Diabetes (NIDDM)
34. Urinary Stress Incontinence

BMI is a mathematical calculation used to determine whether a patient is overweight. BMI is calculated by dividing a person's body weight in kilograms by their height in meters squared (weight [kg.]/height [m]2) or by using the conversion with pounds and inches squared (weight [lbs.]/height [in.]2 x 704.5). This number, however, can be misleading for very muscular people or for pregnant or lactating women.

Obesity increases one's risk of developing conditions such as high blood pressure, diabetes, heart disease, stroke, gall bladder disease and cancer of the breast, prostate and colon.

If maintained, even small weight losses (as little as 10% of body weight) improve your health.

Be not among winebibbers; among riotous eaters of flesh: For the drunkard and the glutton shall come to poverty: and drowsiness shall clothe a man with rags. Proverbs 23:20-21

We Eat Too Much, We Eat The Wrong Foods

A number of different factors have caused us to put on weight. It's more complicated than just "eating too much" (which is exactly what doctors and dieticans believed not too long ago). Weight problems can be the result of glandular malfunction (underactive thyroid, for example) malnutrition, emotional tension, stress, boredom, habit and love of or obsession with food (gluttony).

A major reason for excess weight is poor food choices and malnutrition. We eat too many foods with low nutrient value ("junk food"). These are sometimes called empty calories as they have little or no nutritional value other than the calories they provide. If we cannot use these calories right away, they are readily stored as fat. Refined foods lack most of the nutrients required for efficient energy production and tremendously increase the body's requirement for them. Unrefined foods naturally contain these nutrients. They are lost in processing.

When there is inadequate intake of all essential nutrients, fat is not efficiently burned. Fat is burned only if sufficient energy is produced. Energy production depends on almost every known nutrient.

For example, the B Vitamins are important to produce energy. Fat is burned at a greatly reduced rate if pantothenic acid and protein are under supplied. Vitamin B6 is necessary for the energy conversion of stored fat. It is also a factor in the utilization of protein and fat. Proteins are needed for the proper function of many energy-producing enzymes. Protein cannot be used without other nutrients such as Vitamin B6 and choline.

Vitamin E is needed for fat utilization. Sufficient amounts of E actually double our ability to use fat.

Lecithin aids the cells to burn fat. If we are deficient in the nutrients necessary for production of lecithin (specifically choline and inositol), poor fat utilization results. Instead, the fat is stored.

It's Not Just Counting Calories

Have you ever tried to lose weight by dramatically reducing your caloric intake, and aside from the hunger you experienced, wondered why it was so difficult? In addition to the fact that our metabolism slows when we stop eating or reduce our caloric intake, because you may not giving the body adequate amounts of all of the essential nutrients, especially those needed to burn stored energy (fat), it makes it more difficult.

Malnutrition is one of the major reasons that those dieting have great difficulty losing weight. A diet low in nutritional value rapidly leads to deficiencies. Desserts and sweets require B Vitamins, chromium and many other nutrients in order to be digested and used as energy instead of being stored as fat. Nutritional deficiencies can prevent us from producing enzymes and hormones, which are necessary for the body to even get nutritional benefits from healthy foods eaten. It turns into a viscous cycle.

Consuming more calories than the body can burn off by activities, leads to weight gain. Excess calories are stored in the body as fat. It takes 3,500 excess calories to produce one pound of body fat. That's a lot of calories! This is also how many calories we need to cut back on to lose one pound of body fat.

The number of calories contained in a food will give you a rough idea of its energy value. Just because a food has high calories does not mean it is unhealthy or fattening. Some very healthy, low-fat foods such as beans, rice and whole grains are quite high in calories.

These food are usually high in fiber and complex carbohydrates. For example:

1 cup of canned pinto or kidney beans contains 380 calories, 1 gram fat and 16 grams fiber.

1 cup of cooked steel cut oats contains 220 calories, 1 gram fat and 10 grams fiber.

1 cup of medium grain brown rice contains 218 calories, 1 gram of fat and 6 grams fiber.

1 cup cooked whole wheat pasta contains 220 calories, less than 1 gram of fat and 5 grams fiber.

There is too much emphasis placed on the caloric value of foods. Caloric counts on food labels and calorie charts have little to do with the caloric value to humans. Calorie counts for foods are obtained by burning foods in a bomb calorimeter and measuring the heat produced. These values do not relate to any effects in the human body. The values of four calories per gram for carbohydrates and proteins and nine calories per grams for fat, were developed about 100 years ago. Since then, many people seem to be hung up on the idea of calorie counting and that we should only have "so many" calories per day.

Each individual responds differently to foods as we all have different metabolic rates in our ability to digest and use food. You may know someone who eats a high amount of calories but doesn't seem to gain any weight. This person probably exercises and eats nutrient-dense, low-fat foods like whole-grain cereals, beans, rice, whole-grain pasta, fruits, vegetables, etc.

A great deal of inconsistency exists among listed

caloric values. For example, the caloric value of table sugar mixed with water (such as in sugared sodas or fruit juices) is higher in caloric value and puts on more body fat than table sugar eaten by the spoonful.

Caloric energy from fats are about two and one-half times that of carbohydrates and protein.

The Fat You Eat is the Fat on Your Body!

Fat Calories Are Fatter! Numerous clinical studies show that you put on more body fat by eating fat than by eating the same amount of calories from carbohydrates and protein. There are two reasons for this:

We were created to store fat in preparation for times of food shortages. This was necessary several centuries ago, but today, we should be more concerned with eating too much rather than too little.

The use of body fat for energy is not related to fat intake. For energy, we first burn carbohydrates, then protein and finally fat. It is rare that we actually burn the fats consumed. Most of it, not used for production of hormones, etc. goes directly to storage.

The only fats the body "uses" (are not burned or stored) are the **essential fatty acids (EFAs),** which are <u>unsaturated</u>. Unsaturated fats are needed by the body for numerous biological functions such as the production of prostaglandins and hormones. EFAs are also burned for energy more readily by the body in comparison to saturated fats (usually from animal and dairy products).

The body does not really have any use for saturated fats in any way but to <u>store them</u> – in your thighs, hips, rear, stomach, etc. The fat you eat *is* the fat on your body! Cholesterol is a saturated fat used to produce hormones, but the liver can manufacture all the body needs. Actually, the more cholesterol we eat, the more the liver produces.

Also, although the body can convert excess carbohydrates and proteins to fat, it takes two grams of either to make one gram of fat. The metabolic conversion process uses about a quarter of the calories contained in the excess. So it's a lot of work for the body to convert complex carbohydrate and protein calories to stored fat. You really have to eat a lot of beans and potatoes (without butter and sour cream, of course) before you grow much fat.

Note: Fat cells <u>cannot</u> be changed into muscle cells, they must be <u>burned off by muscle cells.</u> Be very careful of statements made by diet plans or diet products promising to "change fat into muscle." This is impossible.

Avoid Saturated Fats!

Saturated fatty acids are found in animal products (cheese, meat products, eggs, etc.). Unless you are a strict vegan, who consumes no eggs or dairy, it may surprise you to learn how much saturated fat is hiding in your diet. Cut down on saturated fat whenever possible and you'll be healthier and leaner in no time:

- Choose leaner meats and poultry (such as white meat of skinless chicken and turkey).

- Steam, broil or bake foods instead of sauteing or frying.

- Instead of butter, flavor potatoes with fresh pressed garlic, salsa or herbs.

- Instead of donuts, eat bagels, corn bread, English muffins or tortillas. (However, check these for possible high fat content as well.)

- Instead of butter crackers, eat rye crisps, soda crackers, breadsticks - and hold the butter.

- Instead of high fat salad dressing, use non-fat brands, lemon juice or vinegar.

- Use <u>non</u> or <u>low-fat</u> sour cream, cream cheese, etc.

- Instead of ice cream, substitute non-fat frozen yogurt, sherbet, sorbet or ice milk.

- Instead of butter or oil in baked goods, substitute apple sauce or plum sauce.

- Thicken soups with pureed vegetables or beans instead of cream or corn starch.

Avoid Saturated Fat: (% estimate is of total fat.)

Coconut oil/coconut butter *(89% saturated)*

Cream cheese *(64% saturated)*

Hard cheese, i.e. cheddar *(63% saturated)*

Butter *(60% saturated)*

Lamb chops *(54% saturated)*

Beef fat *(50% saturated)*

Palm/palm kernel oil *(46% saturated)*

Pork/bacon *(37% saturated)*

Cottonseed oil *(23% saturated)*

Cholesterol: The Truth

Cholesterol has received a bad reputation in regards to heart health. It turns out that elevated cholesterol levels are not a reliable indicator of heart disease. It is true that cholesterol, because it is a <u>saturated fat</u>, is not exactly healthy. Saturated fat is readily stored and elevated weight does increase one's chances of developing heart disease, as well as many other degenerative conditions. The more fat there is in the body, the higher the production of destructive free radicals through its oxidation. Free radicals are blamed for everything from aging and wrinkles to heart disease.

The body obtains cholesterol in two ways, through the diet and through it's manufacture by the liver, intestines, and all cells in the body. We need cholesterol to make sex hormones, Vitamin D and bile salts. Cholesterol also has a vital role in nerve and brain function.

No matter how much dietary cholesterol we eat, the liver will still go on making it. In fact, a diet high in saturated fats (such as cholesterol) and refined carbohydrates causes an _increase in the body's production of cholesterol._ Because the body produces it, there really is no need to consume it. Vegetarians do very well without it, and actually, have a much lower incidence of weight problems and heart disease.

The following contain dietary cholesterol:

Egg (1 medium) . . . . .274 mg.

Steak (8 oz.) . . . . .208 mg.

Lamb chops (6 oz.) . . . . .168 mg.

Veal cutlet (6 oz.) . . . . .168 mg.

Hamburger (6 oz.) . . . . .162 mg.

Pork chops (6 oz.) . . . . .150 mg.

Ham (6 oz.) . . . . .150 mg.

Ice cream (1 cup) . . . . .59 mg.

Chocolate pudding (1 cup) . . . . . .36 mg.

Whole milk (1 cup) . . . . .33 mg.

Ricotta (1/4 cup) . . . . .32 mg.

Cheddar cheese (1 oz.) . . . . .30 mg.

Mozzarella (1 oz.) . . . . .15 mg.

Butter (1 tsp.) . . . . .12 mg.

Mayonnaise (1 tbsp.) . . . . .9 mg.

Skim milk (1 cup) . . . . .4 mg.

You may be consuming a a lot more fat than you realize. Look at the approximate fat content of the following:

- **One tablespoon butter**
  100 calories/11.5 grams total fat
  7 grams saturated
  31 milligrams cholesterol

- **One 8 oz. glass whole milk**
  244 calories/8 grams total fat
  5 grams saturated
  33 milligrams cholesterol

- **One ounce cheddar cheese**
  114 calories/9.4 grams total fat
  5.98 grams saturated
  30 milligrams cholesterol

- **One ounce cream cheese**
    9 calories/9.89 grams total fat
    6.23 grams saturated
    31 milligrams cholesterol

- **One tablespoon corn oil**
    120 calories/14 grams total fat
    2 grams saturated
    0 cholesterol

- **One tablespoon vegetable shortening**
    115 calories/12.8 grams total fat
    5.2 grams saturated
    0 cholesterol

- **One cup peanuts**
    830 calories/70 grams total fat
    14 grams saturated
    0 cholesterol

- **One 8 ounce T-bone steak**
    800 calories/85 grams total fat
    35 grams saturated
    131 milligrams cholesterol

- **Two ounce (one-eighth pound) bacon**
    315 calories/32 grams total fat
    12 grams saturated
    38 milligrams cholesterol

- **One-third pound chicken**

Dark meat with skin
    125 calories/10 grams total fat
    2.5 grams saturated
    43 milligrams cholesterol

White meat with skin
    72 calories/4.2 grams total fat
    1.3 grams saturated
    29 milligrams cholesterol

WARNING: Fast food restaurants are highly dangerous to your waistline.

There are plenty of restaurants with lots of healthy food choices. Simply select your restaurants carefully, and make educated, careful food selections.

While you may enter a fast food restaurant with good intentions of perhaps ordering a salad with low calorie dressing, the smell of french fries and burgers may convince you to order otherwise. You may instead select one of their other "healthy" or "lean" choices which in reality, are not so lean either.

I have a hard time finding anything healthy in "fast food" places to so avoid them all together (with the rare exception of a few places I know of in southern California - and there may be a few others elsewhere).

	Calories	Fat (g)	% Fat
McDonald's			
Mclean Deluxe w/ Small Fries	540	22	37%
Filet-O-Fish	440	26	53%
Burger King			
Double Whopper w/ Cheese	935	61	59%
Wendy's			
Wendy's Big Classic	570	33	52%
Kentucky Fried Chicken			
Lite'n Crispy Drumsticks (2)	242	14	52%
Hardee's			
Oat Bran Muffin	440	18	37%
Real Lean Deluxe w/ Small Fries	577	18	37%
Big Delux w/Small Fries	730	41	51%

Fats to Avoid

Hydrogenated and partially hydrogenated fats are fats which have been altered from their natural liquid form to become more solid (and stable). This processing alters the natural molecular structure of the fatty acids into an unnatural trans-configuration. These trans-fatty acids are unhealthy and should be avoided. They resemble saturated fats but the body has a much more difficult time processing them. Trans-fatty acids also produce free radicals in the body. Trans-fatty acids are very uncommon in nature, and they are considered by the body to be "foreign."

Trans-fatty acids tend to raise Low Density Lipoprotein or LDL (undesirable) cholesterol levels and lower High Density Lipoprotein or HDL (desirable) cholesterol levels in the blood. In addition, these trans-fatty acids can easily become trapped along arterial walls creating an ideal environment for build-up of plaque and development of atherosclerosis.

In such processing, essential fatty acids are easily destroyed due to the presence of heat, oxygen and light.

Examples of hydrogenated fat products include margarine, margarine-based products, shortening and fats used for frying.

Margarine is Fattier than Butter

In the last 15 years, manufactured fats have replaced cholesterol-raising saturated fats in margarines, snacks and convenience foods.

These partially hydrogenated oils contain damaging trans-fatty acids making them more harmful than the naturally-occurring saturated fats found in butter, other animal-based fats and tropical oils.

Butter contains easy-to-digest, short-chain fatty acids, but relatively few essential fatty acids (only about 2% linoleic acid). Butter also contains about one gram cholesterol per pound.

Butter is more easily metabolized by the body than hydrogenated oils, fats, shortening and margarine. Butter is better for frying, baking and heating because it consists mainly of saturated fats which are relatively stable in the presence of light, heat and oxygen.

Margarine contains altered fatty acids which interfere with the functions of essential fatty acids in the body. Remember, these fatty acids are metabolized much slower than the ones in butter. Margarine and other hydrogenated products are not good for cooking because they are further altered by heat, light and oxygen.

Don't ever believe anyone who tries to tell you that margarine is healthier than butter. **Butter is natural -** the body knows how to process it (in moderation). Margarine is full of trans-fatty acids just waiting to get hung up in your arteries. (Valenzuela) JUST SAY NO TO ALTERED FATS!

Note: Almost all processed foods contain altered fats. Check food labels for hydrogenated or partially hydrogenated oils – and then put if back on the shelf.

Why are Trans-fatty Acids Bad?

Among other results, researchers have found that trans-fatty acids significantly raise LDL cholesterol levels, the bad cholesterol, while lowering the HDL levels, the good cholesterol – even more so than saturated fats. (Valenzuela) In the Framingham Heart Study (a 40-year study covering 5,209 individuals living in Massachusetts) high LDL cholesterol levels combined with low HDL levels was indicative of coronary heart disease risk.

These trans-fatty acids can easily become trapped along arterial walls creating an ideal environment for build-up of plaque and development of atherosclerosis.

Results from other human studies and recent large-scale epidemiologic surveys also clearly show that dietary trans-fatty acids enhance the risk of developing coronary heart diseases. Studies support the idea that lowering current intakes of trans-fatty acids may lower the risk of coronary heart disease. (Nelson GJ)

Other healthier fats are the monounsaturated fats found in avocados, olives and olive oil.

How Much Fat Is OK?

Some nutrition specialists recommend no more than 30% of your total calories should be from fat. For a 2,000-a-day total calorie allowance, this would equal 600 calories per day of fat or 67 grams. This is **much too high**.

The American Heart Association recommends no more than 30 grams of fat per day. This may still be too high if you are trying to lose weight.

If you are trying to lose weight, I suggest consuming no more than 20 grams (countable) of fat per day. This is 180 calories, about 11% of one's total calorie intake.

It is easy to count the number of fat grams you are consuming daily with the new labels on food packages, and there are many great reference books on the market that will give you an idea of the fat content of all kinds of foods, even by brand name.

Dining Out

Be very careful when dining out or ordering take-out. Watch out for foods you think are healthy but turn out to be loaded with fat and/or sodium. Many Chinese dishes, for example, are very high in fat, and as you already saw, oat bran muffins may be loaded with fat too.

Many restaurants have a nutritional analysis available for their menus. Take advantage of these and encourage your favorite restaurants to prepare more healthy choices.

- Avoid rich sauces and "cream of" soups.

- Ask for unbuttered bread and steamed vegetables without butter or sauces.

- Order broiled, baked, steamed or poached foods instead of fried or sauteed.

- Remove all visible fat from meat and skin from poultry before eating.

- Instead of white sauce, stick to red sauce or none.

- Don't stuff yourself. As your stomach expands, so does your appetite. Order smaller portions at a reduced rate or take home one-half for lunch the next day.

CHINESE ENTREES

(1 cup) with 1 cup rice:

	Calories	Fat (g)	% Fat
		(approximate values)	
Sweet and Sour Pork	820	31	34
Kung Pao Chicken	650	23	32
Beef with Broccoli	560	16	26
Orange (Crispy) Beef	725	21	27
1 Egg Roll	190	11	52
Better choices:			
Stir-Fried Vegetables	400	6	14
Szechwan Shrimp	500	8	14
House Lo Mien	500	8	15

ITALIAN ENTREES:

	Calories	Fat (g)	% Fat
Cheese Ravioli (1.5 cups)	625	26	38
Lasagna (2 cups)	958	53	50
Fettuccini Alfredo (2.5 cups)	1,498	97	58
Fried Calamari (1.5 cups)	500	35	61
Better choices			
Linguini w/ Red Clam Sauce (2 cups)	500	13	23
Spaghetti w/Tomato Sauce (2 cups)	490	10	18

Watch Out for Fat in Your Breakfast Cereal!

Approximate fat grams per 1/2 cup serving:

Arrowhead Mills Maple Nut Granola	10
Rainforest Granola	10
Quaker 100% Natural	10
Nature Valley 100% Natural	10
General Mills Raisin Nut Bran	6
Kellogg's Cracklin' Oat Bran	6

Our Sugar Habit

Sugar is much like a drug. It has addictive properties and adverse side effects. Sugar is not a whole natural food that does not even resemble the original sources that God made – sugar cane and sugar beets. Sugar is highly refined, fragmented, denatured and completely stripped of all nutrients which were present in its original form. Sugar cane and sugar beets are natural and contain minerals, vitamins, trace elements, enzymes, essential fatty acids, amino acids and very important FIBER. The final processed result is a pure crystallized form of sucrose, a white "pharmaceutically pure" chemical.

Eating sugar actually creates a loss of essential nutrients (such as B Vitamins and Chromium) which are required to metabolize it in the body. Interestingly, in the processing of raw sugar cane or sugar beets, over 90% of the naturally-occurring chromium is lost. Chromium is needed for insulin to bring glucose into the cells to be used as fuel. Without chromium, we can't burn these calories, so instead they are converted to fat and stored away.

It is not good to eat much honey: so for men to search their own glory is not glory. Proverbs 25:27

When thou sittest to eat with a ruler, Consider diligently him that is before thee; And put a knife to thy throat, If thou be a man given to appetite. Be not desirous of his dainties; Seeing they are deceitful meat. Proverbs 23:1-3

Compared to sugar, honey could practically be considered health food because honey contains several minerals and nutrients to assist in the body's use of the carbohydrate, yet the Bible clearly warns us not to eat too much honey (Proverbs 25:27).

In addition to causing weight problems, sugar is a major contributing factor in the growth of many degenerative conditions, such as diabetes, heart disease, tooth decay, periodontal disease and osteoporosis. Sugar consumption has also been associated with hyperactivity in children and criminal behavior.

Whole foods such as whole grains, vegetables, fruits, etc., are digested slowly and changed into forms of sugar the body can use for energy and for its vital functioning. But refined concentrated sugar is rapidly absorbed into the bloodstream rapidly raising the level of sugar in the blood to a dangerously high level. At this point one will feel an abundance of energy.

The pancreas practically goes into shock in this situation. It over-reacts, dumping an excess amount of insulin into the bloodstream. The body is forced to compensate by producing and releasing high amounts of insulin which allows the sugar to enter the cells so it can be burned.

The excess insulin not only rapidly brings the sugar level down, it lowers it **far below normal**. The term associated with this is **hypoglycemia (or low blood sugar).** When this happens, one can experience a number of unpleasant symptoms such as sleepiness, irritability, headaches, anxiety, insomnia, poor memory, weight gain, sweet cravings, depression, crying spells, cold fingers and toes, blurred vision, dry eyes, etc.

Millions of people suffer from hypoglycemia, many of them unknowingly. Almost everyone, at one time or another, experiences the symptoms of low blood sugar. A diet high in sugar or simple carbohydrates, and also stress, overwork, skipping meals, etc., can trigger the blood sugar level to rise and quickly drop, causing fatigue, headaches, irritability, fainting, blurred eyes, mental confusion, memory lapse, light headedness, etc.

Zinc is closely involved in the body's use of insulin. Zinc is plentiful in the healthy pancreas, where insulin is manufactured and is a constituent of insulin. Individuals with hypoglycemia and/or diabetes are commonly deficient in zinc.

Many adults have poor insulin function. Normal amounts of insulin are produced, but because of the high sugar diet, it is present more often than not. The cells eventually become less sensitive to this continual presence of insulin. Like the first few times the fire alarm goes off, we jump in response to it, but if it continually keeps ringing, we eventually ignore it.

Sugar accounts for approximately 24% of our total caloric intake. On average, we consume over 30 teaspoons of sugar per day per person. Remember, some people consume much less, so that means some people are even taking in **more** than the average.

We realize that candy, desserts and sweets contain sugar, but do you realize how much? Sugar may be found in many places we would not even dream of looking: salt, peanut butter, bread, fruit juices, instant oatmeal, meat products, canned vegetables, mayonnaise, toothpaste, baby food, etc. Many so-called "healthy" breakfast cereals are actually loaded with sugar.

Many manufactures give sugar other names which we may not immediately identify. These include; Corn syrup, corn syrup solids, maple syrup, molasses, cane syrup, fructose, dextrose, maltose, lactose, etc.

Estimated teaspoons of sugar per serving:

Cola beverage (12 oz.) 10
Hard candy (4 oz.) 20
Apple pie (1 slice) 12
Sherbet (1/2 cup) 9
Flavored yogurt (8 oz.) 7
Ice cream (4 oz.) 5
Ketchup (1 tbsp.) 1
Orange marmalade (1 tbsp.) 5
Canned corn (5 oz.) 3

Estimated grams of sugar per serving (1/2-3/4 cup):

General Mills Honey Nut Cheerios 10
General Mills Wheaties Honey Gold 10
Kellogg's Fruitiful or Raisin Bran 9
General Mills Raisin Nut Bran 8
Kellogg's Branbuds 8
Kellogg's Fiberwise 5

Percentage of refined white table sugar by weight:

Non-dairy creamer 60%
Milk chocolate candy 50%
Chocolate cake .36%
Salad dressings . . . . .up to 30%
Yogurt 14%
All Bran 20%
Granola w/ Almonds & Filberts 21%
Lucky Charms 50%
Cocoa Pebbles .54%
Apple Jacks 55%
Sugar Smacks 61%

THE THYROID:

Your Fat Burning Regulator

The thyroid gland regulates metabolism, the rate the body burns calories for energy. Some people feel that their metabolism is sluggish because no matter how little they eat, they just can't seem to lose weight. A high metabolism is given credit for individuals who can eat all day long and not gain an ounce. These individuals seem to have an abundance of energy and can get by with much less sleep than others.

Metabolic or glandular problems may result in weight problems. These may be due to nutritional imbalances: low Vitamin A*, iodine*, zinc, high copper and a number of other contributing reasons. For example, the use and abuse of diet pills forces the metabolism into high gear and is believed to be very hard on the thyroid and also can cause nutritional problems.

* NOTE: If you plan to supplement Vitamin A (daily doses over 50,000 IU) or iodine-containing medications, these should be medically supervised. These can be toxic if taken in excess. Beta carotene or foods <u>containing</u> Vitamin A or iodine are much safer forms to supplement these important nutrients.

Uncontrollable hunger may be due to damaged cells in the hypothalamus (the area of the brain that regulates our desire to eat.) This damage can occur from certain foods, or environmental substances to which one is allergic. Certain medications such as tranquilizers, viral infections, nutritional deficiencies or other brain injuries can also adversely effect this area of the brain.

Hypothyroid

A sluggish thyroid gland can mean a sluggish metabolism. According to Dr. Broda Barnes, many practitioners underestimate the impact of poor thyroid function on the health of the human body. In spite of the relatively small amount of thyroid hormone produced (one teaspoon per year), it is of major importance.

Thyroid hormone is essential to your metabolism and the regulation of fat burning and muscle building. Thyroid hormone directly influences insulin secretion. Animal studies show that low levels of thyroid hormone T3 reduce the insulin response to food. T3 is also essential to prevent catabolism of your own valuable muscle tissue. Remember, burn the fat, keep the muscle!

In the liver, insulin also reacts with another thyroid hormone, T4, which is believed to play a role in the release of insulin-like growth factors, which promote protein (muscle) synthesis.

Many experts maintain that regular laboratory tests are not adequate predictors of the true state of the thyroid. In addition, standard thyroid tests do not isolate the active thyroid hormones, T4 and T3.

Iodine is the major factor regulating production of iodine-containing hormones secreted by the thyroid gland. Iodine deficiency is characterized by obesity, high cholesterol, and coarse hair, and the enlargement of the thyroid gland, called a goiter. Not all individuals with iodine deficiency develop this glandular enlargement. Goiters appear more often in females. Iodine deficiency became less of a problem with the introduction of iodized salt, but deficiencies still exist today. Adult daily requirements are about 150 mcg.

Foods high in iodine may be beneficial to those with thyroid problems. These include:

Amounts are measured in mcg. iodine per 10 grams

Kelp .6,240
Iodized salt 760
Saltwater fish (haddock, herring) . . .33
Catfish .12
Dried beans 12
Seafood .7
Spinach .6
Vegetables 3
Whole grain wheat and oats 1

An under-active thyroid makes it impossible to break down food properly and assimilate nutrients from it. The efficiency of the other glands is also impaired, often severely. Ultimately, every organ, tissue and cell is affected by the output of the thyroid.

Energy is required by every cell in the body. Glandulars provide RNA which the glands use for energy. Glandular RNA is highly beneficial in the special way that it provides energy on a mammal-to-mammal, gland-to-gland basis helping to "tune up" the glandular system of the body.

The pituitary is the master gland. It controls the activity of all other glands in the body. For example, when the body is under stress, the adrenals, the anti-stress glands, have to work over-time. They pull energy from the other glands in the body causing decreased or altered functioning. One may experience loss of sexual desire due to the effects of the gonads, either loss of appetite and weight loss or food cravings and weight gain due to detrimental effects on the thyroid, pancreas or liver.

Tyrosine, an amino acid, aids the conversion of T4 to T3 in the liver and has an important effect on the thyroid.

An Easy Way to Test Your Thyroid and Iodine Levels

Swab a quarter-sized dot of iodine (purchased at any drug store) onto your belly. Check it in 12, 18 and 24 hours. If the stop disappears in 12 or 18 hours, this is an indication of iodine deficiency and suggests that you may benefit from supplementation. If it is still present after 24 hours, your iodine levels are healthy and iodine supplementation is not needed.

NO ONE *LIKES* BEING FAT

For most people, fat and happy really don't go together. Fat and healthy definitely do not go together. No one likes to squeeze themselves into movie seats or airplane chairs, or through the rotating arms while entering a subway or a store. No one enjoys getting stared at while dining in a restaurant or feeling like everyone is thinking "How can she eat that, she's so fat!" No one feels good about putting on a favorite outfit and finding it is too small and uncomfortable to wear any longer. These experiences are probably not on anyone's favorite top 10 list.

But, more serious than these is the greater risk of sickness and death associated with being overweight. This means less time to spend with your family, grandchildren, friends, less time doing the things you really enjoy doing and less enjoyment out of things you once enjoyed.

Added pounds are accompanied by increases in blood pressure, blood fat and blood sugar. Overweight individuals are more prone to cancer (most specifically, breast and endometrial cancer), heart disease, kidney disease, diabetes, high blood pressure, malnutrition, liver disorders, gall bladder disorders, respiratory problems, arthritis, gout, complications of pregnancy, psychological problems and more.

Statistics show that thin people have a longer life span, have more energy and usually feel better than people who are overweight.

Apple or Pear?

One of the most important developments in understanding health risks associated with obesity has come from the two different types of fat distribution; in the the abdominal, upper body region (the apple) or the lower body regions, hips and rear (the pear).

If you are an "apple" (carry most of your body fat in the stomach), you are at a higher risk for developing diabetes or cardiovascular disease (stroke, heart attack, hypertension).

Due to their higher accumulation of abdominal fat, men generally have a higher health risk than women. Overweight women with most fat deposited at the hips and buttocks have a cosmetic problem, but it may not necessarily be a serious health threat.

Several studies have been conducted to understand the relationship between abdominal obesity and diabetes, hypertension and cardiovascular disease. It appears that the increased risk of abdominal obesity is the result of complex hormonal and metabolic interactions. Studies have shown that both total body fatness and the regional distribution of body fat have a significant genetic component. Although abdominal obesity is a significant risk factor for cardiovascular disease, not everyone who is abdominally obese will experience metabolic complications.

High Blood Pressure

Hypertension, or high blood pressure, is primarily caused by a combination of dietary factors and genetics. Obesity is a primary factor of high blood pressure. Achieving ideal body weight has demonstrated to nearly normalize blood pressure of many overweight individuals.

For every 10% weight increase, the blood pressure rises 6.5mm/Hg. Hardening of the arteries and fluid buildup, due to sodium retention or mineral imbalances, are often also associated.

The Sodium-Potassium Problem

The intake of excess sodium is a huge problem, especially in the United States. In the last 100 years, we have experienced a 20-fold increase in our intake of sodium. This was accompanied by about a one-third drop in potassium intake.

In some instances the situation is getting worse instead of better. Many products found in the grocery store such as cheese, soups, frozen dinners, crackers, etc. will reduce their fat content to make the product more appealing to the huge number of diet-conscious consumers. The problem is that with reduced fat, often there is reduced taste, so many manufactures make up for it by increasing the sodium content.

For example:

1 cup whole milk yogurt: **7.5 g. fat/100 mg. sodium.**
The low-fat version: **0.5 g. fat/173 mg. sodium.**

3/4 cup carmel corn: **3 g. fat/30 mg. sodium.**
The light version: **1 g. fat/220 mg. sodium.**

1 tbs. Hellman's Best Mayonnaise: **11 g. fat/80 mg. sodium.** The light version: **5 g. fat/110 mg. sodium.**

2 Aunt Jemima Frozen Waffles: **6 g. fat/410 mg. sodium.**
The light version: **1 g. fat/540 mg. sodium.**

1 ounce shredded part skim mozzarella cheese: **5 g. fat/170 mg. sodium.** The nonfat version: **0 fat/250 mg. sodium.**

We have been so spoiled by eating our potatoes with salt, butter and sour cream, or worse yet, deep fried and salted. It may take a little adjusting as we introduce our taste buds to foods in their natural form, instead of hidden under fat and salt. Soon you won't miss a thing and you will grow to appreciate their real taste.

Obesity and a high salt diet often go hand in hand. High blood pressure is virtually nonexistent in primitive societies that consume diets which are low in salt and high in potassium. The intake of sodium in the form of sodium chloride (table salt) is horrendous. Sodium in this form is difficult for the body to get rid of, and it is easily retained.

High levels of dietary sodium as salt tend to increase losses of potassium and magnesium and possibly some calcium. Physicians have difficulty determining if you have a potassium deficiency because only in extreme cases will the deficiency show up in blood plasma. One must solely rely upon the deficiency symptoms; abdominal bloating, fatigue, mental fuzziness, physical weakness, etc.

In 1988 in a federal health and nutrition survey, people who consumed less than 1,200 mg. (the average intake of potassium) of potassium per day had twice the incidence of hypertension as people who consumed 3,600 mg. per day.

A 12-year-California study showed that an extra 400 mg. of potassium (that's just a glass of orange juice or a generous slice of cantaloupe) daily can reduce risk of stroke-related death by 40%.

Some researchers believe that high potassium levels block the absorption of sodium by the kidneys. Others feel it may act as a diuretic, lowering the volume of blood plasma and thus decreasing blood pressure.

Because of our high salt intake, some experts believe that if there were an DV for potassium, it would be **6,000 mg.**

While we should consume no more than 2,000 mg. sodium per day, the average consumption is probably anywhere from 5,000-15,000 mg. This high amount of sodium increases our losses of potassium. Americans actually consume over four times more salt than the average intake from around the world!

Sodium Chloride Content of Food Items

Salt (1 tsp): **2,132 mg.**

McDonald's Quarter Pounder w/Cheese: **1,150 mg.**

Hardee's Big Country Breakfast: **2,870 mg.**

Hormel Chili (15 oz.): **1,127 mg.**

Tombstone Microwave Pizza, saus./cheese (7.5oz.): **1,300 mg.**

Pizza Hut, Pepperoni Personal Pan Pizza: **1,335 mg.**

Shrimp w/ Garlic Sauce (1 cup) w/ Rice (1 cup): **1,405 mg.**

Cambells Chunky Soups (8 oz.): **822 mg.**

Cambells Chicken Noodle Soup (10 oz.): **1,050 mg.**

Spaghetti with Sausage (2.5 cups): **2,437 mg**.

Linguini with Red Clam Sauce, (3 cups): **2,182 mg.**

Garlic Bread (8 oz.): **1,083 mg**.

Ham (3 oz.) and Swiss (1 oz.) Sandwich: **1,553 mg.**

Kraft Processed American Cheese (2 oz.): **890 mg.**

Green Beans, canned, Del Monte (1 cup): **925 mg.**

Soy Sauce (1 Tbs.):**1,320 mg.**

Dill pickle (1 large):**1,928 mg.**

Keebler Whole Wheat Townhouse Crackers (4): **200 mg**.

Pace Thick and Chunky Salsa (2 Tbs.): **359 mg.**

Cheetos Puffed Balls (1 oz.): **360 mg**.

Aunt Jemima Pancakes w/ Sausage (6 oz) (frozen): **1,140 mg**.

Average for line of frozen meals: **1,175 mg.**

Eat More Foods High in Potassium!

Oranges & orange juice	Bananas
Dates & figs	Avacados
Nectarines & peaches	Potatoes
Chicken breast	Beans & peanuts
Cantaloupe & honeydew melon	Rhubarb

Heart Disease

Cardiovascular disease accounts for approximately 50% of all deaths in the United States. It is estimated that 65 million Americans have some form of heart or blood vessel disease at a cost of over 90 billion dollars a year.

A number of dietary factors have a significant effect on coronary heart disease: Obesity, high cholesterol, high blood pressure and glucose intolerance.

Diabetes

Obesity is associated with a greater risk of diabetes. Diabetes mellitus, whether insulin-dependent or non-insulin dependent, is a disease of carbohydrate metabolism. The majority of those with diabetes have non-insulin dependent type. Many of these individuals are overweight or obese.

For over 50 years we have known that glucose tolerance can be improved by reducing body weight.

Maintaining normal weight is also the primary factor in diabetes prevention. Avoidance of refined sugars not only helps keep your weight down, but it also very simply may prevent diabetes.

Simple carbohydrates in the form of refined sugar are rapidly absorbed into the body causing a rapid increase in blood sugar (glucose). This causes the pancreas to respond with an outpour of insulin to lower the amount of glucose by means of carrying it into the cells to be burned as fuel.

Natural unrefined foods such as grains, beans,

vegetables, etc. contain fiber which has a slowing effect upon absorption rate. Complex carbohydrates take longer to break down into simple sugars and thus cause a more gradual release into the blood stream. This is far less stressful to the pancreas.

Liver Damage

Liver problems are common among overweight persons, largely because of a diet high in fat. The liver has the responsibility to metabolize the fat we eat. If it becomes overloaded, fat will accumulate in the liver tissue impairing its 500 other important functions such as producing all kinds of enzymes, bile and hemoglobin, processing glucose, proteins, vitamins and most other compounds used by the body. The liver is also responsible for metabolizing the alcohol, nicotine and any other poisons we ingest from our water, food or air.

A diet including complete proteins, the B Complex Vitamins, choline, Vitamins B12, C and E and lecithin aid the restoration of the liver.

Varicose Veins, Hemorrhoids, Hiatal Hernias, etc.

Varicose veins (unsightly, sometimes painful, distended veins usually seen in the legs) are commonly seen among individuals who are overweight. The excess weight is strenuous on the lower part of the body which must carry the weight around.

Constipation commonly accompanies a high fat,

low fiber diet. The straining to pass stools is implicated as a cause of varicose veins, hemorrhoids and hiatal hernias. When you strain to pass your stools, high pressure is placed upon the abdominal cavity. These pressures are transmitted to the veins draining the lower limb. The pressures are held back at the first set of valves in the leg veins. Eventually, these valves give way from the top down, causing the unsightly bulging veins.

Hemorrhoids are engorgements of normal blood vessels in the rectum. Continual straining to pass stools forces blood to engorge the hemorrhoidal vessels.

This increased pressure on the abdomen may also contribute to hiatal hernia, a condition in which part of the stomach is pushed upward through the diaphragm into the chest cavity. This also may contribute to heart burn.

Other health problems associated with being overweight include: **Gout**, which is associated with a fatty diet, **Gall stones**, which are formed by cholesterol and bile which are not carried out of the body by fiber, **Arthritis** and **Gynecological Irregularities.**

EAT LESS, LIVE LONGER

Low Calorie Diets Prove Healthful

According to Roy Walford, researcher and author of *The 120-Year Diet*, we could plan on living 30 to 50 years longer than we originally expected if we consumed less calories, a lot less calories.

A number of studies have shown that the life span of animals can be extended by restricting their food intake. Rats fed 40% fewer calories lived 50% longer than their unrestricted peers. That corresponds to humans living to be 150-160 years old.

Walford and a number of others have shown that cutting calories in young animals delays a loss of heart muscle function that ordinarily occurs with aging, and can extend the reproductive years. Fewer calories keep their immune systems from deteriorating with age.

Walford and associates reported in the 1992 Proceeding for The National Academy of Sciences that a calorically restricted (average of 1,780 kcal./day), low-fat (10% of calories), nutrient-dense diet in humans has a large number of health benefits. The diet significantly lowers weight in men and women, lowers blood glucose, lowers total leukocyte count, reduces cholesterol levels and decreases blood pressure.

Skinny People Die at the Slowest Rates!

William Castelli, director of the famous Framingham Heart Study which monitored the health of thousands of residents of the city near Boston since 1958, reports that in Framingham, Massachusetts, those who weigh between 11-20% below the average weight for their height have the lowest risk of early death. Other researchers have also demonstrated the effect of caloric restriction on age-associated cancers.

Enhanced Immune Response

Animal studies show that low-calorie diets have a positive effect upon immunity. Walford and his associates demonstrated that dietary restriction enhanced immunity to an infectious agent, influenza, as well as enhanced other immunologic parameters. Dietary restriction significantly inhibited the normal age-related decline in immune responses.

Enhanced Use of Insulin

Walford and other researchers also investigated the relationship of aging and restriction of dietary calories upon insulin. In this study, they found that reducing calories by 52% extends maximum life span by approximately 33% and increases insulin receptors by 15% to 25%. Increased insulin receptors allow us to more efficiently use the energy from the food we eat.

Reduced dietary calories, enhanced nutrient intakes and modification of fatty acid composition of serum lipids have demonstrated to benefit patients with non-insulin-dependent diabetes mellitus (NIDDM) in a study with 86 obese subjects (aged 40-64) with recently diagnosed NIDDM.

In this study, the patients undergoing dietary therapy resulted in greater weight loss, better metabolic control and an improved blood lipid profile than the control group.

While many diabetics are aware of the need to limit simple sugars, most do not limit their intake of dietary fat or increase their intake of high fiber foods, which are also necessary to obtain ideal weight and stable blood sugar levels.

Free Radical Protection

Oxidation is part of the natural metabolic process of the body. When fatty acids are burned as fuel for the body, oxidation occurs, which produces free radicals. In humans the level of oxidative DNA damage can be lessened by caloric restriction and dietary composition. Less food eaten means less oxidation and fewer free radicals produced. (Simic)

The basic mechanisms of aging and its retardation by caloric restriction remain unclear. Reducing calories may retard aging based on the reduced production of mitochondrial free radicals. (Feuers) The less food we consume, the less work it is for the body to process and metabolize it – burning calories produces free radicals.

Improved Inflammatory Conditions

Inflammatory conditions such as arthritis, psoriasis, allergies, etc., are very difficult to treat successfully. Imbalances of inflammatory and anti-inflammatory hormones contribute to the problem. Caloric restriction may help reduce production of a powerful inflammatory component (Interleukin-6 or IL-6) in the body. Blood levels of IL-6 are normally very low – usually non-detectable in the absence of inflammation. As we grow older, however, the levels increase. (Ershler)

Researchers also speculate that IL-6 may contribute to the development of several degenerative diseases that are common in late-life including arthritis, lymphoma, osteoporosis and Alzheimer's disease. This age-related process can be largely prevented by life span-extending dietary restriction. (Ershler)

Reduce Risk Factors for Heart Disease

Weight Loss Helps Manage High Blood Pressure

Your reason for wanting to lose weight may be as simple as wanting to look and feel better, but the actual results of weight loss expand much further. Obesity is a risk factor for the development of heart disease. We know weight reduction is an effective long-term therapy for maintaining normal blood pressure. (Davis)

Researchers (Singh and associates) found that dietary strategies are highly effective in reducing other risk factors associated with cardiovascular diseases. To study the role of diet in cardiovascular-risk-factor intervention, 458 high-risk individuals were asked to eat a cardiovaso-protective diet. Such a diet is high in complex carbohydrates, vegetable protein, fiber, Vitamin C, potassium and magnesium. Fats consumed consist largely of polyunsaturated fats, avoiding saturated fat and cholesterol. Total fat intake should make up about 20% of the total caloric intake.

After one year, there was a significant decrease in total risk factors:

1. **Significant reduction in blood cholesterol**

2. **Reduced blood pressure**

3. **Reduced weight and modification of other risk factors and complications in patients with risk factors of coronary heart disease**

Fast Food, Gluttony and Sin?

An interesting article, *Is eating on the run is as big a sin as gluttony?* by Janet Street-Porter, author of *Coast To Coast,* examines common eating habits.

She points out that *Italy's Catholic bishops declares that fast food is anti-Catholic and that the act of eating it undermines fundamental Christian values* and states that *the humble hamburger is lacking the community spirit of sharing. It seems that eating on the run is as big a sin as gluttony (eating too much).*

Fast food too often means eating quickly so you can rush off and do other things....Let us not confuse the consumption of fast food with the experience of eating a meal together with friends or family. While the popularity cooking programmes increases on television, our cooking skills atrophy and sales of ready-cooked meals soar. The time when the family shares a meal at the end of each day is ending. No one seems willing to take the time to prepare healthy meals for their family... Our poor health and weight problems show it.

THE PROBLEM WITH MOST DIETS...

Only 5% of those dieting to achieve permanent weight loss will be successful and reap the associated health benefits. This leaves 95% unsuccessful. The health implications of failed weight loss attempts are numerous and include negative effects on both physical and psychological well-being.

Instead of "dieting," it is far better to take small, positive, enjoyable steps toward healthy eating, active living and a positive self-image.

There are a number of problems with the way we diet and try to lose weight. There is a great deal of misinformation about losing weight. When we say we want to "lose weight," we really mean that we want to "lose excess body fat." If we also desire to tone or build muscle, the number on the scale may not change or may even increase, while we look and feel smaller and more compact.

3 Main Problems with Popular Diet Programs:

1. They concentrate on total body weight, rather than body fat.

2. They tend to reduce vital muscle which is the major body component which burns fat. The more muscle you have the easier it is to burn fat.

3. *They aim at rapid weight loss, which causes the rate of metabolism to slow down and fat preservation to occur.*

4. *They do not teach healthy eating habits that can be maintained for a lifetime. When you go off "the diet" and return to your old eating habits, the weight you lost will quickly be regained.*

Fad diets which tell you to eat only the specified foods and liquid diets have serious flaws. As soon as you return to eating and drinking normal amounts of calories and essential nutrients, most of the weight you suffered so much to lose is regained.

Many studies have shown that the weight loss programs available are simply ineffective for long term ideal weight maintenance.

One scientific study at Syracuse University compared three different groups of overweight women using three different weight loss programs used by commercial diet centers. One group was put on an 800 calorie diet. The second and third groups were on an 800 and 1,200 calorie diet, respectively, and were also given "behavior therapy," the popular counseling support offered by centers such as Weight Watchers.

All groups rapidly lost weight. The group on 800 calories plus behavior therapy, lost the most. Over 90% of the women in this group lost more than 20 pounds.

However, within a year, almost half of the women in all three groups gained it all back. Within five years,

81% had gained it all back and **more.** The women in the behavior therapy group were the least successful at keeping the weight off compared to the others. *(Report of National Institute of Health Expert Panel of Weight Loss. Bethesda, MD, 1982.)*

Americans are spending an estimated 33-36 billion dollars on weight loss supplements and programs. Not bad for the economy, terrible on our pocketbooks.

Dieting Dangers

The desire to lose weight is often accompanied by irregular eating habits, meal skipping, etc. Frequently, this leads to cravings and unstable blood sugar levels. To satisfy these cravings, too often, individuals eat sugars and simple carbohydrates, instead of complex carbohydrates, protein and satisfying, nutritious whole foods. These empty-calorie foods, in the long run, intensify cravings. In addition, these extra, empty calories eventually mean excess stores of fat.

High protein/Low carbohydrate diets are designed to quickly deplete the body's supply of carbohydrates, after which, fat stores are burned for energy. Breads, pastas and sweets are traded for eggs, cheese, bacon and other fatty foods. These diets have helped many people lose weight, but it is extremely hard on the liver, and cannot be maintained long term. When individuals go back to their old eating habits, the weight comes right back on.

Very low calorie diets, starvation diets and rapid weight loss put too much stress on the body and are very dangerous to health. This can cause electrolyte imbalances, abnormal heart rhythm (arrhythmias), heart attack and sudden death.

This is a major concern for obese people using starvation or semistarvation diets for weight reduction. There have been numerous reports of sudden death due to ventricular arrhythmias of the heart.

Obesity is associated with cardiovascular changes and abnormalities. With weight loss, the mass of the heart and left ventricle decrease, but some signs of left ventricular dysfunction remain. Health effects of weight loss appear to depend upon diet duration and upon whether protein and mineral nutritional status is maintained. Copper, potassium and magnesium deficiencies may play important roles in promoting an electrically unstable heart.

Stress, by eliciting imbalance, may act upon an electrically unstable heart to provoke problems.

Weight loss reduces many of the health hazards associated with obesity including insulin resistance, diabetes mellitus, hypertension, dyslipidemia, sleep apnea, hypoxemia and hypercapnia and osteoarthritis. Potential adverse effects of weight loss include a greater risk for gallstone formation and cholecystitis, excessive loss of lean body mass, water and electrolyte problems, mild liver dysfunction and elevated uric acid levels. Less consequential problems such as diarrhea, constipation, hair loss and cold intolerance may also occur. These temporary adverse effects are not severe enough to indicate that one should not attempt weight loss, nor do they outweigh the benefits of permanent weight loss. (Pi-Sunyer FX)

Yo-Yo Dieting

Yo-yo dieting refers to the situation where a person repeatedly loses and gains weight. This is not only frustrating, it is very unhealthy. In spite of the fact that you probably feel like you are constantly dieting, you are actually getting fatter. Each time one loses and gains, the body percentage of <u>fat increases</u> and the percentage of lean muscle decreases. Also, one tends to gain more weight each time, with decreasing ability to get as low as you were before. This is very damaging to health.

Fad diets (Scarsdale Diet, Grapefruit Diet, Watermelon Diet, Beverly Hills Diet, Hollywood Diet, many various liquid diets, etc.) which promote rapid weight loss, often referred to as crash dieting, should be avoided because they can be very dangerous.

Studies at the Department of Food Science at Rutgers University analyzed a number of "the best of the diet books;" Pritikin, Atkins, the California, Stillman, Scarsdale, The F-Plan, I Love America Diet, Carbohydrate Cravers and others, and found that they were all seriously deficient in vitamins, minerals and fiber.

Losing weight rapidly is not the best way to lose fat and not the best way to **keep it off**. Many fad diets cause a very impressive and rapid initial loss of weight, while there is relatively little loss of fat compared to the loss of electrolytes. You want to lose fat, *not* minerals, other nutrients or muscle tissue.

Sudden weight loss can damage the heart, gastrointestinal tract and metabolism. Food, nutrient and caloric restrictions also make one more susceptible to illness and infection.

As soon as you return to eating and drinking normal amounts of calories and essential nutrients, most of the weight you suffered so much to lose is regained.

Losing Fat Vs Losing Muscle

Nutrition scientists tells us that low calorie diets (consisting of 800-1,200 calories daily) cause a tremendous loss of muscle tissue. Of the weight lost, up to 45% comes from loss of muscle. *(Oskai)*

Many super thin women existing on 400-800 calories per day, may measure 30% body fat. The ideal range for women is between 15-20%. The average is actually about 22%. Female athletes generally are between 16 -18%. The amount of fat considered essential for women is 12%. Essential means that women cannot go lower than this level without impairing health and athletic ability.

The ideal range for fat percentage is much lower for men, 10-14%. Only 3% is considered essential.

Body fat composition can be determined in several ways. Bipolar electrolysis is the most accurate. Other methods include underwater weighing, infrared light machine and the pinch fold test which have about +/- 2% accuracy.

Very low calorie diets of 400 to 800 kcal/day appear attractive as they generally show weight loss of 1.5 to 2.0 kg/week compared to 0.2 to 0.5 kg/week found with the traditional diet.

When very low calorie diets were first becoming popular, intake of quality protein was not stressed. The result of this was about 60 deaths, many of which were attributed to loss of lean body mass and in particular, cardiac muscle atrophy. Exercise can help slow the depletion of lean body mass during very low calorie diets, but medical supervision is strongly advised if you decide to pursue this type of serious dieting.

Dangerous Drugs

All drugs are dangerous. We are all too familiar with the Phen-Fen fiasco a few years back and in November of 2000, the FDA (Food and Drug Administration) alerted the public of the dangers of another drug which has been used for sometime as an appetite suppressant, phenylpropanolamine (PPA).

PPA is found in popular over-the-counter weight loss pills and also some brands of cough syrup, cold and allergy medications. Some of the manufactures of these medications have issued voluntary withdrawals of these products because of the increased risk of seizures and hemorrhagic stroke (bleeding in brain) among individuals (especially women) who use them.

PPA also has a number of dangerous side effects on the heart and the kidneys. It increases blood pressure, can cause nausea and heart palpitations and can be highly addictive. Teenage girls are especially susceptible to cardiac abnormalities induced by PPA, even after only a minimal overdose. (Chin)

Weight loss associated with the use of PPA is very stressful to the body and is not permanent. When the weight returns, the percentage of body fat is higher than before dieting. This can turn into a vicious cycle until the problem is corrected with proper diet.

Currently, the FDA still allows benzphetamine (dexedrine amphetamines or "speed") to be sold in weight-loss products as an appetite suppressant. Its use is accompanied by restlessness, insomnia, rapid heart beat, increased blood pressure and dry mouth. For those who perhaps need to lose weight the most, it is highly dangerous. It is contraindicated for those with arteriosclerosis, cardiovascular disease and high blood pressure, as well as glaucoma and over-active thyroid.

Dehydration

Diuretic use among those wishing to shed a few pounds has been going on for years. Diuretics work by altering hormone levels triggering the kidneys to work faster, actually **forcing** water from the body. Because **more** than just "excess" water is eliminated, valuable mineral electrolytes are lost and homeostasis in the body is upset. Users may become more and more dependent on the drugs, demanding higher doses to get the same effect. Eventually, some may not be able to urinate without them.

Used long term, diuretics can mess up one's hormone levels leading to loss of control of body water distribution and swelling, especially of the legs.

The same principal of using and abusing diuretics applies to laxatives. Dependency is easy to develop and difficult to correct. Laxatives interfere with absorption of minerals and Vitamin D.

Eating disorders such as anorexia and bulimia are common, especially among high school and college-age women. The combination of bulimia and drug abuse is also very common in women. Drugs frequently abused include diuretics, emetics (causes vomiting), laxatives, and diet pills, as well as alcohol, cigarettes, speed, cocaine and other illicit street drugs.

Natural Diuretics

Bloating and water retention is a very common complaint among individuals who want to lose weight. Natural products which help eliminate excess water are superior to drugs because they **do not force** water out of the body.

Kelp, a natural health-giving sea vegetable, is rich in protein, iodine, magnesium, and calcium. Kelp is often used in conjunction with Vitamin B-6 (pyridoxine), which is a natural diuretic.

Other natural mild diuretics include parsley, buchu, uva ursi, juniper berries, dandelion leaf, couch-grass, watercress, watermelon seeds, asparagus and azuki (or aduki) beans.

Uva Ursi is an especially good antiseptic for bladder and kidney infections.

Don't forget water, the best, safest, natural diuretic of all! Drink at least eight large glasses every day!

FIBER

Your Staple to Reaching and Maintaining Your Weight Goal

Fiber is a carbohydrate food component which is not digested and broken down as are other carbohydrates, or proteins and fats. Fiber passes through the stomach to the small and large intestine, virtually unchanged. Its major constituents are cellulose, lignin and pectins.

Fiber contains no calories. It provides us with no energy or nutritional value. Its value lies in what the fiber does while it is in the body.

Dietary patterns have changed dramatically over the last century. Modernization and processing continue to increase the distance between a natural food and the food on the table. You may know that granulated sugar is in most cases derived from sugar cane. But do you know what sugar cane actually looks like?

Why is it that the farther away a food moves from its natural state, devoid of fiber, or of any nutritional value whatsoever, the more marketable it becomes?

The more a food is processed, the more profitable it is for the manufacturer: Did you know that a pound of baking potatoes may cost $0.35 a pound, but you would have to pay $4.20 for a pound of potato chips?

Many common health problems are linked to our

intake of fiber, or actually, **LACK** of it. Denis Burkitt, M.D., the man who achieved fame for identifying and curing the first human cancer caused by a virus (now known as Burkitt's Lymphoma), took interest in the differences in American and African dietary patterns and the differences in health problems.

During the 20 years when Dr. Burkitt practiced surgery in Africa, he noticed that the people there did not suffer from the disease conditions which were popular in Western civilization. Appendicitis, coronary heart disease, obesity, gall stones, varicose veins, hemorrhoids, colorectal cancer, hiatal hernia and other common Western problems among Africans and other societies not yet polluted with Western culture, occurred perhaps less than 1 in 100, 300 or even 500 times compared to the incidences in the U.S. or Europe.

Burkitt came to the conclusion that these diseases must be preventable, and if they are, why are we spending our time treating them? We should be preventing them.

Burkitt came to the conclusion that fiber was a critical factor followed by refined sugar and white flour. Burkitt was not the first person on the fiber bandwagon. Hippocrates used whole grains as medical treatments, and the Kellogg brothers have been pushing the health benefits of cereal grains for almost a century.

Wherever Westernization of dietary habits travels, disease follows. Obesity is first seen, followed by diabetes, appendicitis, gallstones, heart disease and so on. Constipation would be nonexistent if we would eat foods in their natural state before processing.

About two centuries ago, the refining of grains began. Now cereal fiber is a rarity, instead of the norm. If you want to purchase real whole grain cereals such as millet, rye, buckwheat, wheat, flax or amaranth, you usually have to go to a special health food store. Most whole wheat breads are soft, airy white breads with a little wheat bran added for color. Real whole grain bread is very dense, weighing probably 3 or 4 times more than soft white bread.

Effect of Fiber on Insulin

Removing fiber from a naturally high carbohydrate food, dumps too much sugar into your blood stream, causing production of too much insulin. The job of insulin is to "take" the glucose into the cells to be burned for energy. Too much insulin initiates an enzyme to tell our brain that there is too much glucose, and the ability of the liver to store any excess is exceeded. The remaining glucose is stored as fat.

Removing fiber (for example, when you squeezed an orange to produce orange juice), allows the carbohydrates to rapidly convert into simple sugars and to quickly enter the bloodstream. The pancreas releases a larger amount of insulin to compensate. The insulin triggers the enzyme to tell the body to start storing all that excess glucose.

It is far better to eat the whole orange, than just drink the juice, and throw away the fiber. You will notice how much fuller you feel after eating a whole apple compared to drinking a glass of apple juice.

A 100 gram apple is, in a way, 98 grams apple juice held together by 2 grams of fiber.

Betty Kaman, New Facts about Fiber

As fiber travels through the digestive tract it takes with it fat debris from the intestinal tract that would otherwise contribute to weight gain and formation of excess gasses.

In the colon, fiber holds onto water, which helps form a softer, larger, more consistent bowel movement. Fiber also carries bile and fat out of the body. Without fiber, much of this fat is reabsorbed and recirculated through the body.

By helping cleanse fat and debris from the digestive tract, nitrogen and sulphur gasses are also reduced, allowing for more optimal absorption of important nutrients, including oxygen, which increases the metabolic rate in the body and is important for memory and energy levels.

Bile Breaks Down Fat

The name bile doesn't sound very appealing, but bile acids are actually a very good thing. They break down fats and in the presence of fiber, latch on to it and exit the body.

Bile is produced in your liver and stored in your gall bladder until needed. It is made from cholesterol, and when it leaves the body, it rids the body of its raw material.

Types of Fiber

There are several kinds of fiber, all of which are beneficial for various effects on the body.

Lignins, Cellulose and Hemicellulose are structural insoluble fibers. Oats and barley are rich sources of cellulose. Flax is a rich source of lignins.

Hemicellulose is broken down by fermentive bacteria in the colon more readily than cellulose is broken down. Hemicellulose has tremendous water-holding abilities. Psyllium husks are an example of hemicellulose.

Pectin is a gel-forming natural substance (used as a thickener in jam and jelly) contained in all fruits and vegetables. Pectin is lost in the refining process. Pectins change from an insoluble fiber in unripe fruit to a soluble fiber in ripened fruit. Pectin does not alter transit time. Soluble fibers are fermented by colonic bacteria to a much greater extent than insoluble fibers.

Pectins used for nutritional supplements are commonly derived from apples, lemons and carrots.

While the National Cancer Institute recommends that adults consume 25-30 grams of fiber daily, the average American diet provides only about 11 grams.

Gums, sometimes called mucilage, are not part of the structure fiber of plants, but are indigestible and so are considered a water-soluble dietary fiber. Gums are commonly derived from the Locust bean, guar, agar-agar and carrageenin.

Different fiber sources have different effects on the intestinal tract. The effects of soluble fiber, such as psyllium husks, are different than the effects of insoluble fiber such as wheat bran. Both types are important and necessary for good health.

Soluble Fiber

- Lowers cholesterol
- Reduces heart disease risk
- Improves blood sugar, lowers blood pressure
- Promotes growth of friendly flora

Insoluble Fiber

- Aids digestion
- Aids elimination
- Promotes regularity
- Contributes to bowel cleansing (natural laxative effect)

Fiber Content in Foods:

Highest to Lowest

1. **Whole grain cereals** - whole grain wheat, rice, corn, barley, rye, buckwheat, millet, oats, amaranth and flax

2. **Legumes** - peas, beans, lentils
   Nuts
   Seeds
   Dried fruits

3. **Root vegetables** - potatoes, yams, kohlrabi, carrots, parsnips, turnips, beets

4. **Fruits**
   Leafy vegetables - lettuce, cabbage, celery

5. **Animal products** contain no fiber- beef, chicken, fish and other meats, eggs, milk and milk products (cheese, yogurt, etc.)

Benefits of a High Fiber Diet

The health benefits of a high-fiber diet are too numerous to list. Fiber is simply a necessary dietary component which really went unnoticed until we started suffering the effects of eating a diet without it.

One fiber study for the treatment of obesity and hypercholesterolemia demonstrated how just the daily addition of 15 grams (2 teaspoons) of a high fiber food supplement could result in a significant weight loss and also a drop in blood cholesterol levels. (Kaul)

Weight Loss Benefits of Fiber:

- Fiber helps you feel full and eat less.

- Fiber holds water and increases fecal bulk.

- Fiber binds bile acids carrying them (and fats) out of the body.

- Fiber reduces or normalizes transit time. (The time it takes for the food to travel from the mouth to the elimination channels.)

- Fiber causes fermentation in the large bowel (it provides something for the bacteria to grow upon.)

- Fiber helps fight constipation and bloating.

- Fiber improves colon health by "keeping things moving."

- Fiber helps eliminate toxins and waste products faster.

- Fiber lowers the risk of colon-rectal cancer – the second leading cause of death in this country.

- Fiber reduces elevated cholesterol.

- Fiber lowers risk of heart disease – the leading cause of death in this country.

- Fiber is a natural, inexpensive approach to health and longevity.

Transit Time

Transit time is the period it takes for food to travel from the mouth until its waste products exit the body. The longer it takes, the more time is available for reactions to occur amongst the waste materials. This putrification can lead to unhealthy waste products, including the production of carcinogenic substances. These residues can even be reabsorbed into the blood stream causing problems with metabolism and other complications.

You can check your digestive transit time yourself. Swallow a few kernels of whole corn without chewing. Transit time varies with the food you consume so continue to eat the foods you normally do. Watch to see how long it takes for the corn to appear in your stool. ***A healthy normal range would be between 12-20 hours.***

If it takes less than 10 hours, there may not have been adequate time for proper digestion and assimilation of the nutrients in your food. The exception to this would be if you are already consuming a very high fiber diet and the stools are well formed, not loose.

If it takes longer than 24 hours, you can consider yourself constipated and it would be very wise to consume more fiber and drink more water. Variation of transit times can range from 47 to 123 hours in the same person, depending on diet, drugs and fluid intake.

A wonderful thing about fiber is that it helps normalize the digestive tract whether it is working too slow or too fast.

While the average transit time for young healthy adults in Western countries is an unbelievable three days, in Third World countries, average transit time is less than 18 hours. You don't see colon cancer in these countries.

In the United States, the number of people who are constipated is larger than the number with normal transit time. Among the elderly, some individuals do not pass a bowel movement for as many as 14 days.

Constipation is not only uncomfortable, it is very unhealthy. Toxins from fermenting waste products can be reabsorbed in the blood stream, creating all sorts of problems ranging from fatigue to colon cancer. Bacteria react with bile salts to form carcinogens. Colon cancer is the second most common form of cancer.

A supplement containing a range of natural fibers including various grains plus fruit fibers is probably more effective compared to a single fiber supplemented alone.

The Power of Synergism

It is far better to consume something in combination with other factors for a synergistic effect rather than isolated from its natural source and taken alone, such as psyllium husks, or the bran of grains. Oat bran is beneficial, but it is better to eat the whole oat, than just the bran.

In nature, nothing exists in isolation. You won't find ascorbic acid or magnesium growing on a tree somewhere.

One of the recommendations of the National

Cancer Institute is to eat a variety of fruits and vegetables, but they also should have added, "and utilize the entire fruit or vegetable."

Whole Foods

Nature has a plan for everything. The whole basis behind nature is for everything to work together... nothing in isolation...to use everything to its full potential, wasting nothing.

A more natural diet satisfies hunger because it satisfies the body's real hunger for nutrition.

Processing removes components of a food which the body needs to use that particular food to its fullest extent. There are many examples we can use to further demonstrate:

• Eggs contain fat in the form of cholesterol, but also contain lecithin to help you emulsify and use the fat.

• Fruits and vegetables should not be peeled because they contain vitamins, trace minerals, bioflavonoids and many other important trace components, many of which may not even be identified yet. (Buy organic to avoid pesticide residue.)

• Most fruits (and many vegetables) are high in sugar, but the fiber they contain slows down their absorption into the bloodstream preventing too much insulin from being released. It is far better to eat a raw, whole piece of fruit, than to just drink the juice and throw away the fiber.

• Some antioxidants have shown to be more beneficial when consumed in their whole food form compared to high doses of an isolate in the form of a supplement.

It is well known that fruits and vegetables high in beta carotene offer a protective effect against cancer and some other degenerative diseases. But it is now realized that there is more to the secret than just <u>beta</u> carotene. Beta carotene is just one of dozens of different types of carotenes found in foods. It is now believed that large amounts of just <u>one</u> form (as in a high potency supplement) can interfere with absorption, transport or use of other forms, causing health problems. (Albanes)

• Vitamin E also has a number of different naturally occurring forms, It seems that high doses of Alpha-tocopherol may not be such a good idea for cancer protection after all. Because of its cardioprotective effects, a low dose supplement is advisable, no more than 100 mg. daily, and stick with **mixed tocopherols.** (Albanes)

Flax Seed

Flax seed is an excellent whole food high in fiber. It is rich in very important nutritional components which are otherwise hard to find: lignins, a cancer-fighting fiber and also the Omega 3 essential fatty acids (linolenic). Flax seed contains approximately 60% linolenic acid (LNA), and is probably the best source of Omega 3. It also contains the other essential fatty acids, 16% Linoleic (Omega 6), and 18% Oleic (Omega 9).

Flax seeds are also an excellent source of soluble lignin fiber. Flax seed lignins have a very solid amount of research demonstrating their anti-cancer effects, specifically uterine, cervical and breast cancer. Other research has demonstrated the ability of flax seed lignins to reduce blood lipids by as much as 27%. (Cunnane)

Other nutrients provided by flax seed include Vitamin E, beta carotene, calcium, magnesium, manganese and potassium. Flax seeds also contain high quality protein.

What to do with freshly ground flax seed:

- Mix with non-fat yogurt, cottage cheese, cheese dips, etc. (the fiber helps the body rid itself of fat, especially saturated fats found in many dairy products).

- Mix into meat loaf, meat balls, soy balls, etc.

- Mix into homemade breads, waffles, muffins or other baked goods.

- Sprinkle onto salads, scrambled eggs, breakfast cereal (hot or cold), rice or steamed vegetables.

- Blend into protein or fruit shakes.

The fatty acids in flax seed are highly susceptible to destruction and rancidity by exposure to heat, light and oxygen. This is why it is important to use flax freshly ground. Try to prepare an amount which can be consumed right away and refrigerate any unused portions as soon as possible.

FOODS TO SUPPRESS HUNGER

Nothing is more important in a successful weight control program than learning to control hunger. Appetite begins in the brain. When blood sugar is low the brain produces neurotransmitters which tell you you are hungry. Your brain decides what to eat. Each food we eat effects us in a different way. Some foods are more satisfying (to our hunger) than others. An apple may be more satisfying than a chocolate chip cookie, even though they have approximately the same number of calories. Sometimes you can eat something, feel satisfied and then be hungry again in 10 minutes.

When you eat, as your blood sugar rises, insulin is released telling the cells to start burning off the glucose. Some foods cause the blood sugar level to increase more quickly and to a higher level than others. A dramatic rise in blood sugar corresponds to a dramatic rise in insulin and a rapid fall of glucose.

Low insulin levels promote calorie and fat burning.

Elevated insulin levels:

1. Stimulate the appetite.

2. Cause blood sugar to fall rapidly and to very low levels causing fatigue, irritability and more hunger.

3. Cause fewer calories to be burned and more to be stored as fat.

71

Glycemic Index

Glycemic index is a rating system indicating how different foods effect the rise in blood sugar. Foods which have such a dramatic effect on blood sugar are rated higher. Reactions are compared to table sugar, which is rated 100, which has the most dramatic effect of sugar levels.

Eat more low glycemic index foods which promote a slow, moderate rise in blood sugar and insulin after eating them. This helps keep hunger in check and encourage the body to dissolve body fat by converting it into energy. These foods allow you to consume more calories without gaining weight. They actually increase your metabolic rate.

Avoid High glycemic index foods which cause sudden, unstable swings in blood sugar, first with rapid, very high sugar and insulin surges, followed by a crash of sugar to excessively low levels. These foods increase your cravings for simple carbohydrates, sweets, etc., causing overeating and binging.

• Increase foods high in soluble fiber such as lentils and beans, which have a lower glycemic response.

• Fat lowers the glycemic rating because it slows absorption. Ice cream and yogurt, for example, which are high in sugar, have a lower glycemic rate because of their high fat content. Reduced fat and non-fat varieties have much higher glycemic index rates.

• Juiced and pureed fruits and vegetables produce a higher glycemic rating than the whole fruit or vegetable.

• Generally, the longer you cook foods like potatoes or vegetables, which are primarily carbohydrates, the more simple the sugars become and the higher the glycemic rating.

• The more you alter a food (through processing), the higher the glycemic index rating becomes. Mashed potatoes have a higher rate than whole potatoes. Rice flour has a higher rate than whole rice. The more intact (natural) the food is, the more healthy your insulin response will be after eating it.

High Glycemic Index Foods:
Avoid these foods to minimize insulin increases!

GLYCEMIC INDEX

Sugar	100
Rice, instant	91
Carrot juice	90
Honey	87
Corn Flakes & similar ready-to-eat cereals	85
Rice Krispies	82
Dried figs	80
White rice	80
Vanilla wafers	77
White bread or bagel (plain)	75
Cheerios	74
Watermelon	72
Saltine crackers	72
White potatoes	70
Raisins	68
Angel food cake	67
Grapenuts cereal	67
Cream of wheat cereal	66
Oatmeal - quick cooking	66
Banana	65

Low Glycemic Index Foods:
Eat More of These Foods!

Soybeans	.15
Fructose	.20
Cherries	.22
Barley	.22
Plums	.24
Grapefruit	.25
Lentils	.25
Kidney beans	.27
Pasta (protein enriched)	.28
Split peas	.32
Strawberries	.32
Apples	.30
Apricots, dried	.30
Chickpeas	.36
Oranges and pears	.36
Whole wheat spaghetti	.38
Navy beans	.38
Yogurt	.38
Spaghetti pasta	.40
Apple juice	.41
Grapes	.43
All Bran cereal	.44
Rice, parboiled	.47
Sweet potatoes	.48
Pumpernickel bread	.49
Oatmeal - regular	.50

(steel cut oats would probably be around 40 or less)

Some Excellent Food Choices:

Apples

An Apple a Day... is no joke!

National health authorities recommend we eat at least five servings of fruits and vegetables daily to obtain the benefits of the fiber and nutrients they contain. These nutrients in fruits and vegetables can strengthen the body's defense against cancer and other major diseases. Apples contain just 80 calories, no sodium, cholesterol or saturated fat.

Apples contain numerous important beneficial vitamins, minerals, fiber, enzymes, etc. Apples and apple juice contain phenolic compounds shown to help reduce cholesterol. These antioxidants protect against oxidation of LDL (low-density lipoproteins), the "bad" cholesterol that clogs arteries. Eating apples not only lowers cholesterol, it also improves the ratio of beneficial high-density lipoproteins (HDL) to harmful LDL.

Research also indicates that D-glucaric acid, an ingredient in apples, may be a natural regulator of cholesterol. A diet rich in D-glucaric acid can help reduce damaging LDL by up to 35%.

Apples are an excellent source of pectin, a soluble fiber found in most fruits and vegetables also shown to help reduce cholesterol.

Apples are a delicious source of dietary fiber which helps digestion and promotes weight loss. They are filling and satisfying making delicious snack and dessert food that's good for you. A medium apple contains about five grams of fiber, more than most cereals. If you travel, apples are easy to carry with you to eat for lunch – eliminating the need to stop somewhere "dangerous" to eat.

Beans and Lentils

Beans and lentils are inexpensive, but hold valuable health benefits. They are an excellent source of protein, yet unlike most other protein sources, have virtually no fat. Lentils, cow peas, black, fava, kidney, lima, pinto and white beans all contain less than one gram of fat per one-half cup (cooked) serving.

Surprisingly, soy beans contain nine grams of fat per one-half cup (cooked) serving. This fat is largely unsaturated so it is still a far better source of protein compared to animal products which are rich in saturated fat. Soy beans are very high in fiber, containing 4-5 grams per serving.

Beans are mineral-rich too, containing potassium, iron, calcium, magnesium and others.

Beans come in many different colors, sizes and even shapes, but nutritionally they all have wonderful affects, especially on cholesterol, due to their high content of soluble fiber. Studies show that adding one cup of cooked beans to the daily diet can reduce cholesterol levels by 19%. (Anderson) The insoluble fiber in lentils and beans promotes digestive health.

Note: If you feel that beans give you gas, be sure to chew them well. Chewing is very important because digestion of carbohydrates starts with the digestive enzymes in the mouth. To some extent, the more work you do in the mouth, the less work the rest of the digestive system has to do!

Also, make sure that your beans are cooked well. Start with easier-to-digest legumes such as lentils and peas. The more you eat, the easier it will become for your digestive system to digest them. Lastly, adding a small amount of baking soda into the water as they cook helps reduce such digestive complaints.

Oats

One of the simplest and best things you can do for your body is to eat a bowl of steel cut oats for breakfast at least five mornings a week. Steel cut oats is the least processed way to consume oats. Oat meal is more highly processed and instant oats are the worst because they also add sugar and other chemicals we do not need. You can increase variety by adding raisins, chopped apple, orange rind, cinnamon, cardamom or other things.

Oats (and also barley) are rich in the complex carbohydrate fiber known as beta glucan. Research shows that this substance regulates blood sugar so is excellent for those who are diabetic or hypoglycemic. (Wood, Wursch, Tappy)

Beta glucan is also an excellent immune system stimulant. It increases levels of white blood cells and encourages them to work harder to clean up debris and pathogens in the body. There is also evidence showing its ability to help us fight cancer and tumors. (Hoffman, Ito, Ross)

There is also research showing beta glucan helps regulate our cholesterol levels. (Uusitupa, Braaten, Lia, Bobek, Behall, Lovegrove)

Recommended low-fat, fiber and nutrient-rich foods to help curb hunger:

Apples

Amaranth

Avocados (the fat is mostly monounsaturated and they are very high in fiber)

Barley

Beets

Beans (all varieties)

Broccoli

Bulgur

Cabbage

Guava

Mushrooms (fresh)

Oats - steel cut

Peas

Soy

Squash (all varieties)

Turnips and turnip greens

Wheat bran

Vegetables - fresh and raw especially

WEIGHT LOSS SUPPLEMENTS

When looking for an effective weight-loss product, one can get more than confused with all the advertising claims that manufacturers are making these days. Even breakfast cereals are claiming to help us *"keep the muscle, lose the fat."* Trying to figure out which products are effective is also frustrating and can be expensive.

Alfalfa

This is one of the richest food sources of vitamins and minerals. The minerals are in a balanced form which promotes absorption. Alfalfa provides a rich supply of fiber providing a natural stool softening effect.

Alfalfa also contains high amounts of chlorophyll, a natural detoxicant which helps cleanse the body of toxins. This combined with the fiber makes it an excellent food or supplement for those trying to lose weight.

In addition, alfalfa contains saponins. These help prevent the absorption of dietary fat through the stomach and intestinal wall. This substance has shown to actually remove cholesterol from the blood stream. Even better, it reduces dangerous LDL cholesterol and increases levels of beneficial HDL cholesterol.

Suggested daily intake: 4-6 500 mg. tablets each meal.

Apple Cider Vinegar

Apple cider vinegar contains maltic acid, a natural component of apples, which helps stimulate the body's digestive processes. Apple cider vinegar encourages the elimination of excess fluids and bloating and help stimulate metabolism.

Because it is fermented, the vinegar joins with the alkaline elements and minerals in the body to produce "cell scrubbing" action. Apple cider vinegar is rich in potassium, a mineral which creates an antiseptic quality in fat-burdened cells. It stimulates the metabolism and accelerates oxidation required to get rid of fats.

Apple cider vinegar is available in a number of formulas, usually in a tablet form, while some people prefer to drink it straight. Years ago, the KLB-6 Diet™ became popular where apple cider vinegar is often combined with kelp, lecithin and Vitamin B-6.

Bran

This is an inexpensive form of fiber which provides bulk, improves digestion and elimination. Fiber removes fat from the body, lowers cholesterol and slows sugar absorption. When sugar levels raise too high too fast, insulin levels raise which causes storage of sugar in the form of fat. Also, you will feel hungry again sooner. Also, remember to drink extra water if you are increasing fiber to avoid constipation. Bran may be obtained from oats, wheat, rice or other cereal grains. It is better to use the whole grain in food preparation.

Suggested daily intake: 36-50 grams daily (food and supplements combined).

Branch Chain Amino Acids

This group of amino acids including **leucine, isoleucine** and **valine** are valuable to maintain energy and muscle tone if you are trying to lose weight. These amino acids are necessary to build and maintain muscle tissue. If the diet provides inadequate protein, the body may be forced to metabolize muscle tissue protein for energy.

Suggested daily intake: 100-500 mg. of each.

Bromelain

This enzyme derived from raw pineapple digests protein making amino acids available for formation of muscle tissue. The more muscle you have the easier it is to burn fat and to prevent fat storage.

L-Carnitine

Carnitine is a nonessential amino acid which may prove to be indispensable to people who want to lose weight. Carnitine's value lies in its ability to stimulate the burning of fat cells for energy. Carnitine can be made by the body if the raw materials (methionine and lysine in the presence of Vitamin C) are present.

L-Carnitine, and also inositol and choline, are lipotropic factors which assist and promote an increase in the body's ability to convert fat stores into energy by increasing fat burning capabilities.

Suggested daily intake: 500 mg. twice daily.

Chitosan

Chitosan, a naturally-occurring polysaccharide derived from the exoskeleton of shellfish, such as shrimp or crab, is chemically similar to the plant fiber, cellulose. It provides bulk and assists in the elimination of toxic wastes. Chitosan has the unique ability to significantly bind to fats acting as a "fat sponge" in the digestive tract. Chitosan is a positively-charged fiber molecule which is magnetically attracted to negatively-charged fat molecules. Clinical studies show chitosan can bind up to five times its weight in fat.

Chromium

Chromium, an essential trace mineral, is naturally found in carbohydrates such as cereals, grains and natural sugar. At least 90% of the chromium (along with other nutrients), is removed in the refining process. Chromium is not among the few nutrients added back in during "enrichment." Chromium deficiencies are very common and contribute to insulin dysfunction.

The diets of nine out of 10 people lack chromium! The recommended daily intake for chromium is about 120 mcg., yet about 60% of the people in one study received less than half of this amount. (Anderson)

Chromium deficiency increases fat production because it slows the burning of food for energy. Food which is not burned is stored as fat. (Anderson)

The body requires chromium to use carbohydrates as energy. Chromium is needed for insulin do its job, as a "door keeper" that controls the passage of nutrients and other important compounds through the walls of the 70 trillion cells in the body. These cells need glucose to burn for energy, but if the glucose can't get in, it can't be burned. Instead, the glucose is stored and converted to fat.

Insulin is crucial for the control of hunger, energy production, fat burning, muscle building and cholesterol utilization. Chromium can help insulin do all these things better!

A high-sugar diet increases chromium excretion 10 to 300%. Exercise and physical work requires chromium and thus depletes stores faster. If you exercise on a regular basis, your daily requirement for this mineral may be many times higher than someone who is sedentary.

You do not have to be diabetic to experience some of the symptoms of mild insulin dysfunction:

1. Fatigue   **2. Sugar cravings**
3. Fat production   **4. High cholesterol levels**

Chromium Spares Protein

Muscle cells play a crucial role towards one's ability to maintain an elevated metabolic rate as they are the ones burning the glucose for energy. The more muscle you have, the more calories you can consume without gaining fat. When trying to shed excess pounds, you certainly want to hold onto that muscle, and just lose fat. Chromium helps us do that!

Insulin directly stimulates protein synthesis and retards protein breakdown in muscles (Kimball, Fukugawa). This protein sparing effect of insulin tends to decline during low calorie diets as insulin levels decline, which results in loss of muscle and organ tissue.

By "sensitizing" muscle to insulin, supplementing chromium helps preserve muscle in dieters so that they "burn" more fat and less muscle. (Hasten)

At the San Antonio Weight Loss Clinic, it was demonstrated that <u>one does not even have to exercise to benefit from taking chromium picolinate</u>. Without exercise and without dieting, the chromium picolinate group lost 4.2 lbs of fat and gained 1.4 lbs of muscle tissue. (Kaats)

The best results were experienced by older individuals, which is not surprising because chromium deficiency increases with age. <u>Those taking 400 mcg. daily had better results than those taking 200 mcg. daily.</u> (Kaats)

DHEA

Dehydroepiandrosterone (DHEA) is a hormone that readily converts into testosterone (the "male" hormone) and has many other important affects in the body.

DHEA speeds up metabolism. Animal studies suggest that DHEA may be very effective in treating obesity as it speeds up the metabolism (Yen), decreases the number of fat cells in lean rats and decreases the number and size of fat cells in obese rats. (Cleary)

DHEA reduces gluconeogenesis, the process where the body converts stored glycogen to glucose so that it can be burned by the body for energy. Excess calories are converted to glycogen in the liver and stored to be burned later when needed. Obesity and diabetes are characterized by high levels of glucose occurring in spite of increased levels of insulin.

Insulin instructs glucose to enter the cells to be burned (oxidized) for energy. In both insulin resistant mutant mice and in normal aging mice, DHEA increases sensitivity to insulin, thereby potentiating its effects of increasing metabolism or glucose burning. (Coleman) In this way, DHEA helps *burn* those excess calories *instead* of storing them as glycogen.

DHEA reduces the desire to eat. A recent study in diabetes prone rats indicates that one of DHEA's weight reducing mechanisms may operate through the increase of serotonin levels in the hypothalamus region of the brain, thereby increasing the release of cholecystokinin, the satiation hormone. This hormone reduces one's desire for food by creating a feeling of "fullness." DHEA fed rats showed an increase in serotonin levels in the hypothalamus. This was associated with increased activity of this satiation hormone which reduced food intake and lowered body fat. DHEA's affects on satiation may also be related to its beneficial regulatory effects on insulin and blood sugar.

DHEA prevents fat storage/Increases fat metabolism. DHEA produces lipid and insulin-lowering affects.

High doses of DHEA (encapsulated) were given to five normal weight males at a dose of 1,500 mg. per day divided into four doses. After 28 days, with diet and physical activity remaining normal, four of the five exhibited a mean body fat decrease of 31% with no overall weight change. At the same time, the LDL levels fell by 7.5% which protects them against cardiovascular disease. (Nestler)

A study on DHEA and visceral fat accumulation (fat surrounding the internal organs in the body) in relation to sex hormones in obese men and women undergoing weight loss therapy, showed a correlation among women, but not men. The study included 70 healthy obese men and premenopausal women, aged 27-51, on a diet for 13 weeks.

In women, an abundance of visceral fat was significantly associated with diminished levels of sex hormone-binding globulin and free beta-estradiol/free testosterone ratio and to elevated levels of free testosterone. Loss of visceral fat was significantly related to rises in the sex hormone-binding globulin level and the free 17 beta-estradiol/free testosterone ratio independent of total fat loss. In obese men, sex steroid levels appear not to depend on the amount of visceral fat. (Leenen)

DHEA is not without side effects, especially when taken in high amounts and especially in women. Side effects include heart palpitations (rapid heart beat), acne, facial hair (women), irritability/anxiety, headaches and sleep disruption. Individuals experiencing such side effects should reduce their dosage.

To help reduce side effects, a liquid sublingual is the preferred delivery system for DHEA. Pregnenolone, the precursor to DHEA can also be used, however, because the conversion to testosterone is less, the weight loss/fat loss effects are not as dramatic.

Essential Fatty Acids

Essential Fatty Acids (EFAs), especially the Omega 3's, EPA and DHA are important for weight loss. They are needed to produce hormones and other substances that regulate metabolism and break down fats. These fats are used by the body, not burned or stored like saturated and monounsaturated fats.

Primary sources include flax seed and fatty fish such as salmon and cod. If these are not part of your daily diet, you should consider supplementing.

Suggested intake: 2,000-6,000 grams daily.

Fiber

Popular fiber supplements include **Cascara Sagrada, Chitosan, Guar Gum, Glucomannan, Flax Seed, Alfalfa, Pectins** (from grapefruit and apple) and **Psyllium Husks**. Most of these are covered individually.

Garcinia Cambogia

Garcinia cambogia, HCA or (-)-Hydroxycitric acid is a fruit extract with a chemical composition similar to citric acid (the primary acid in citrus fruits). Preliminary research, based on laboratory experiments and animal research, suggests that HCA may be a useful weight loss aid. (Lowenstein, Triscari) HCA has been demonstrated in the laboratory (but not yet in trials with people) to reduce the conversion of carbohydrates into stored fat by inhibiting certain enzyme processes. (Cheema-Dhadli, Sullivan) Animal research indicates that HCA suppresses appetite and induces weight loss. (Sullivan) One case report found that eating one gram of the fruit containing HCA before each meal resulted in the loss of one pound per day. (Sergio)

HCA is found in only a few plants, with the richest source being the rind of a little pumpkin-shaped fruit called Garcinia cambogia, native to Southeast Asia. Thai and Indian cuisines use this fruit (also called Malabar tamarind) as a condiment in dishes such as curry.

The optimal intake level of HCA remains unknown. Although dieters sometimes take 500 mg. of HCA three times per day (before each meal), this amount is far below the levels used in animal research (figured on a per-pound body weight basis). The effect of HCA is enhanced when used in conjuncture with a low-fat diet, because HCA does nothing to reduce the caloric effects of dietary fat. There were no well-known drug interactions with Hydroxycitric acid.

Glucomannan

Glucomannan is a polysaccharide (many simple sugars) containing mannose and glucose. It is also a soluble fiber and can absorb up to 200 times its weight in water. Asian women have claimed for years that it helps them maintain a desired weight.

Glucomannan reduces blood fats, discourages weight gain, helps to keep blood sugar levels normal and relieves constipation. When ingested, it takes on a jelly-like consistency and expands to make the stomach feel full. This helps reduce overeating.

Glucomannan also acts as a bulking agent in the colon, which stimulates peristalsis (the muscular movement that causes bowel evacuation).

Clinical studies confirm that glucomannan in konjac tubers lowers both total cholesterol and LDL cholesterol – without affecting diastolic blood pressure. When given to obese children, konjac glucomannan (KG) decreased cholesterol and triglyceride levels significantly, without any negative effects. Obese adults who took one gram KG with eight ounces of water one hour before meals three times a day for eight weeks reported an average weight loss of 5.5 pounds, and overall reductions in total cholesterol and LDL.

In one double-blind trial, ten days of treatment

with KG returned the bowel habits of patients with chronic constipation to normal. Another study showed that patients given either three-four grams daily noted an average increase of three and six more bowel movements per week, respectively, without additional diarrhea or flatulence.

Konjac glucomannan helps keep glucose at optimal levels, suggesting that KG may help control glucose levels in diabetics. When used along with conventional treatment, KG not only helped normalize and maintain blood sugar levels in patients with type 2 diabetes, it also lowered both cholesterol and systolic blood pressure.

Experimental studies also indicate that KG may protect against certain types of cancer. When elderly people are given glucomannan, the bacteria in the gut changes and encourages the growth of the "friendly bacteria" such as Bifidobacterium. This is associated with a reduction in pro-cancerous nitrosamines, proteins thought to be responsible for the development of liver cancer and other cancers. Good bacteria also encourages peristalsis that leads to a bowel movement. This helps move waste products out of the body before they can promote cancer or other illnesses.

Glucomannan supplements may reduce the absorption of Vitamin E and other fat soluble vitamins. This may be due to enhanced bile activity, which speeds the evacuation of fats from the body. It's not unusual for supplements that alter blood lipid status to have an effect on fat-soluble vitamins, but you need to be aware of this so you can supplement accordingly.

Aloe vera also contains glucomannan. Aloin is the cathartic anthraquinone laxative that causes bitter aloe – the medicinal preparation of aloe that is used for constipation, not burns – to trigger painful intestinal cramping. Konjac and konjac glucomannan do not contain aloin, and do not have this uncomfortable effect.

Glutamine

This is an amino acid which is useful for the control of carbohydrate cravings. For someone who craves carbohydrates the first thing they reach for is sweets, cookies, bars, chips and french fries, instead of the complex carbohydrates we should be eating.

Suggest daily intake: 500 mg. three times daily.

GLA (Gamma Linolenic Acid)

GLA, a polyunsaturated essential fatty acid, promotes cholesterol normalization and is a precursor to prostaglandin hormone compounds which stimulate energy production and calorie burning. GLA is a type of linolenic acid, an essential fatty acid, which we require daily because the body cannot make it.

Brown fat, which is believed to be the most metabolically active fat in the body, can be encouraged to burn up more fat with GLA. GLA has been shown to stimulate the brown fat and boost the body's use of its fat stores.

Guar Gum

Watch out for supplements containing high amounts of this fiber. It works by absorbing water, adding bulk, but it has fatally blocked the throat and intestines of some people. Many substances don't work well in isolation, and in this case, can be very dangerous.

Gum Guggul

This fiber-like derivative comes from an Indian herb Commiphora mukul. Studies show that gum guggul effectively helps lower elevated cholesterol and triglyceride levels. It has shown to be very safe, even in obese individuals.

Iodine

Iodine is the major factor regulating production of iodine-containing thyroid hormones. Iodine deficiency is characterized by obesity, high cholesterol, coarse hair and the enlargement of the thyroid gland, called a goiter. Not all individuals with iodine deficiency develop this glandular enlargement. Goiters appear more often in females. Iodine deficiency became less of a problem with the introduction of iodized salt, but deficiencies still exist today. Adult daily requirements are about 150 mcg.

A sluggish thyroid gland can mean sluggish metabolism. Thyroid hormone is essential to your metabolism and the regulation of fat burning and muscle building. Thyroid hormone directly influences insulin secretion. Low levels of thyroid hormone T3 increase insulin resistance - the reduced response by cells to insulin to burn glucose. (Glucose which is not burned is stored and converted to fat). T3 is also essential to prevent catabolism of your own valuable muscle tissue.

In the liver, insulin also reacts with the thyroid hormone, T4, which is believed to play a role in the release of insulin-like growth factors, promoting protein (muscle) synthesis.

One indication of a sluggish thyroid may be feeling cold all the time. You can also check your temperature in the morning when you wake up, before getting out of bed. If it is below 98 degrees consistently, for several days, you may have a sluggish thyroid.

Kelp

Kelp is a seaweed that is rich in vitamins, minerals and many trace elements. It contains significant natural iodine and has been used in the treatment of thyroid problems. Iodine is important for the production of thyroid hormone which is involved in regulation of metabolism and rate of "fat burning" in the body.

Licorice

Licorice is known as "The Great Detoxifier" in China. This herb is widely used to support the health of the adrenal glands and is believed to prolong the life and increase the effectiveness of the adrenal hormones. It is believed to do this by helping to maintain electrolyte balance in the tissues and thus preventing their destruction. (Card) Licorice is also anti-inflammatory and aids the immune system by stimulating the production of interferon. (Abe)

Liver Glandulars

The liver is the principal site for fat metabolism of the body. Any nutrients which support the liver are of benefit to the dieter. Liver concentrated supplements will boost energy production through enhancement of glucose metabolism.

Phenylalanine

This amino acid suppresses the appetite by stimulating the neurotransmitters in the brain that control our appetite. Phenylalanine stimulates our other appetites and desires. It is often used for depression because it boosts the antidepressant neurotransmitters in the brain.

Suggested intake: 500 mg. two times daily.

Phosphatidylcholine (PC)

This lipotropic is naturally found in lecithin, which is found in soy and egg yolks. It is a main source of choline which is essential to the formation of the neurotransmitter acetylcholine. Choline also helps metabolize fats and is needed for optimal liver functioning. Choline deficiency results in impaired release of fats resulting in accumulated fats.

Potassium

This mineral works with sodium to regulate the body's water balance and normalize heart rhythms. Potassium works inside the cells, sodium works outside. It helps dispose of body wastes and increases energy. Diuretics, alcohol, coffee (and other caffeine sources) and sugar flush potassium out of the body. A deficiency will result in bloating and water retention.

A great deal of potassium is lost in the processing of foods and deficiencies are prevalent. If you exercise, and you should be, you need more potassium.

Suggested intake: 500 mg. two times daily.

Pyruvate

Pyruvate (in the form pyruvic acid) is created in the body during the metabolism of carbohydrates and protein. Pyruvate may aid weight loss efforts. (Stanko) A clinical trial found that pyruvate supplements enhance weight loss and also result in a greater reduction of body fat in overweight adults consuming a low-fat diet compared with placebo. (Stanko) Animal studies suggest that pyruvate encourages weight loss by increasing the resting metabolic rate in overweight individuals. (Ivy)

Preliminary research indicates that pyruvate functions as an antioxidant, inhibiting the production of harmful free radicals. (Deboer, Cicalese) Preliminary research with animals suggests that due to its potential antioxidant function, pyruvate may inhibit the growth of cancer tumors. (Stanko)

In addition to being formed in the body during digestive processes, pyruvate is present in several foods, including red apples, cheese, dark beer and red wine. Pyruvate is also available as a supplement.

Most human research with pyruvate and weight loss has used at least 30 grams per day, which is a very high amount – around 30 capsules. Be wary of supplements that contain or recommend less than this as there is no evidence that taking less than this amount would have any weight loss effects.

High intakes of pyruvate can trigger gastrointestinal upset, such as gas, bloating and diarrhea.

Spirulina

Spirulina is a blue-green algae renowned for its high usable protein content (65%), which also contains a high concentration of vitamins, minerals, essential fatty acids and other special nutrients. It is especially high in beta carotene, as well as numerous other carotenes, Vitamin B-12 and the other B Complex Vitamins, iron, essential trace minerals and gamma linolenic acid (GLA), an essential fatty acid.

As a protein source, it is more concentrated than any other natural food and contains all essential amino acids (fish and meat contain 15-25%, soybeans contain 35%, dried milk contains 35%, peanuts contain 35%, and eggs contain 12%). Spirulina also contains many valuable non-essential amino acids. The protein content is easily digested and assimilated in the body.

GLA, a polyunsaturated essential fatty acid, promotes cholesterol normalization (Becker) and is a precursor to prostaglandin hormone compounds. These hormones stimulate energy production, and therefore are very important for fat metabolism. Prostaglandins also boost the effectiveness of insulin.

St. John's Wort

The herb St. John's Wort interrupts depression-binge eating-cycle by helping improve mood. As a serotonin reuptake inhibitor (SRI), it increases serotonin levels which are necessary for the satiety response of the brain. Without serotonin, one continues to eat (especially triggered by depression) long after they normally would "feel full."

5-HTP (Tryptophan precursor)

This amino acid precusor helps curb cravings for carbohydrates, especially sweets. Most overeating is simply compulsive, thoughtless eating. Suppression of appetite, then, should focus on the brain. 5-HTP can also alleviate insomnia which is common among those trying to lose weight.

Suggested intake: 100 to 300 mg. daily.

Tyrosine

This amino acid (with another amino acid, phenylalanine) is needed to form the hormones, adrenaline and noreadrenaline. Adrenaline encourages the breakdown of stored fat. Noreadrenaline is a neurotransmitter that promotes mental alertness, memory, and suppresses the appetite.

Tyrosine is also needed to form serotonin and dopamine, neurotransmitters which also help one feel full and satisfied. Studies show increasing serotonin levels can help one reduce carbohydrate cravings.

Studies have shown that dopamine deficiencies are common among obese individuals. (Wang)

Vitamin B-6

Vitamin B-6 (pyridoxine) is necessary for proper assimilation of protein and carbohydrates. It acts as a natural diuretic to encourage the elimination of excess fluids and bloating.

Thermogenics

Cutting back on caloric intake causes the body to slow down the rate at which it burns calories, making it more difficult to lose weight and causing one to feel tired and sluggish. You can safely boost your metabolic rate through natural thermogenic substances. Thermogenics refers to increased production of energy or heat in the body. They promote burning of stored fat, and help maintain muscle tissue. Natural herbal stimulants can also help you feel energetic and alert.

Some studies support the idea that reduced energy expenditure (slow metabolism rate) is common among overweight individuals and a risk factor for the development of obesity. (Donner, Goran)

Coleus Forskohlii

Coleus forskohlii is an Aryvedic herb and member of the mint family. It is the only known plant source of diterpene forskolin. This compound enhances adenylate cyclase, an enzyme that increases AMP production as part of the Krebs/ATP energy cycle. AMP causes a biological chain of reactions in the body that paces metabolism and food-induced metabolism, and provides mechanisms for controlling body composition and lean body mass. Forskolin may be involved in the regulation of insulin and also may stimulate thyroid action.

Studies show that 25 mg. of forskolin twice daily can improve overall body weight by increasing lean body mass and by decreasing weight from body fat. (Badmaev)

Guarana

Guarana is a famous Brazilian herb used for centuries for its natural stimulants such as theobromine, theophylline and caffeine. (da Fonseca and Salvadori) Guarana works synergistically with other thermogenics such as **Ma Huang** and **White Willow**, making their fat burning effect stronger when used together.

Ma Huang

Chinese herbal Ma Huang which contains natural ephedrine has been safely used for three thousand years. It decreases appetite and its thermogenic effects prevent slowing of a resting metabolic rate even while one reduces their caloric intake. (Pasquali)

Studies demonstrate that the ephedrine/caffeine combination is even more effective in improving and maintaining weight loss, further, it saves lean body mass. Used properly, the dangers and side effects are minor. (Toubro)

Ma Huang is a classic sympathomimetic agent. It works by stimulating beta-receptors throughout the body. Stimulating beta-receptors on brown adipose tissue (BAT) cells, causes them to burn white fat cells for energy at a faster rate. Chronic stimulation of these receptors seems to cause BAT cells to proliferate, explaining why thermogenic agents become more effective when you use them for an extended time. (Astrup)

Stimulating beta-receptors also results in brochodilation which is why Ma Huang has been so useful for treating asthma and respiratory problems.

Siberian Ginseng

Siberian Ginseng is probably the most highly regarded tonic herb in the world. Its active components include saponins which are restorative and thermogenic. (Kumar)

Its popularity for anti-stress, anti-fatigue, continues to grow. Taken alone it does not necessarily provide "quick energy" like some of the other "stimulant" herbs, but in a blend its remarkable properties are enhanced.

Used on a daily basis, Siberian Ginseng strengthens the body's adrenal-corticol system to gradually build up your body's ability to resist stress and fatigue. In older individuals, Ginseng influences cellular enzyme activity promoting a strengthening effect on the heart and brain resulting in increased vitality and quality of life. (Caso)

Gota Kola

This Asian tonic herb is excellent for strengthening of the adrenal glands. It is often used in combination with Ginseng as they work well together, but they do not have the same action. It does not have as much research behind it to understand its effects to the extent that we do Ginseng. We do not understand how this herb provides its energizing effects as they are not derived from caffeine-like compounds that are contained in Guarana or Ma-Huang. Kola Nut (which also contains caffeine) is sometimes confused with Gota Kola, but they are not the same.

Ginger

This root commonly used in cooking and baking produces a generalized stimulatory effect in the digestive tract which gently energizes the blood. Some people actually report a feeling of warmness throughout the body. When taken in combination with other herbs or nutrients, Ginger hastens their delivery into the blood stream. This not only increases circulation and energy. it also stimulates the vasomotor and respiratory centers in the central nervous system.

While Ginger does not have a direct effect on blood sugar, it is highly recommended for hypoglycemics. Ginger is known for digestive system and anti-morning sickness affects, but it also reduces inflammation, pain, cholesterol levels and platelet aggregation.

Bladderwrack

Bladderwrack is an edible seaweed similar to the more widely known kelp. These are popular foods throughout Asia. They are rich in iodine and other trace minerals. Bladderwrack has mild thermogenic properties, is a natural diuretic and is considered one of the best weight-reduction plants available.

Brindall Berry

Brindall berry fruit contains Hydroxycitrate acids, which is a natural thermogenic, appetite suppressant (Hellerstein) and is a potent inhibitor of the ATP citrate lyase enzyme. This enzyme is required for the formation of fats in the body tissues. (Hildebrandt) Many studies demonstrate that by inhibiting this enzyme, hydroxycitrate can reduce body fat accumulation, due in large part to a reduction in appetite. (McCarty)

Exercise is a great way to burn stored fat as it increases the amount of glucose required to meet the increased demands of the body. As liver glycogen stores decline, fat stores will be converted and burned for energy. Prior to exercise, administration of hydroxycitrate, may aid endurance by promoting gluconeogenesis. Researchers state that chromium may further potentiate this activity. (McCarty)

Rehmannia Root

This Chinese herb is derived from a plant similar to Ma-Huang. It has weak thermogenic and diuretic properties. (Lewis) It is useful to purify the blood and to strengthen the heart and kidneys by eliminating excess acids in the body.

Yohimbine

This is a plant substance derived from the bark of the African tree Pausinyslalia yohimbe. Yohimbine blocks alpha-2 adrenergic receptors, part of the sympathetic nervous system. When activated alpha-2 receptors block the burning of fat. By preventing the activation of these receptors, yohimbine seems to help maintain the burning of fat. Unlike beta-2 agonists (caffeine, Ma Huang, PPA, etc.), yohimbine helps burn stored fat without affecting heart rate or blood pressure.

The amino acid tyramine, and foods containing high amounts of tyramine (aged cheese, red wine and beer), should be avoided if one is taking yohimbine. Together they may cause high blood pressure and other complications.

Water

Water, in sufficient quantities, plays a major role in helping to control weight. Water is, in fact, the most important nutrient, because we cannot live more than three to fours days without it.

Water accounts for over two-thirds of our total body weight. In overweight individuals, it may be even more. The reason for obesity-related fluid storage involves insulin, salt and water retention. If you feel you are retaining water - drink more! Water is a natural diuretic. If you are not consuming enough water daily, the cells will hold onto it and may cause you to feel bloated when you are actually dehydrated.

We lose water through perspiration and respiration, but the biggest loss occurs through urine to flush out body waste. The feces also contain a large amount of water. All this water has to be replaced - every single day.

Water improves digestion and makes you feel full. A big glass of water can be used for sipping instead of snacks while watching television or while working.

Water and fiber are very important components of healthy weight loss. Many toxins are stored in our fat cells. As we burn these cells, as is the goal when losing weight, these toxins are released. If there is adequate amounts of fiber in the body, the fiber will help to pull these toxins out of the body before they can cause problems elsewhere. Like fiber, water is important to keep the contents of the bowels moving.

Suggested intake: Eight large glasses daily.

EXERCISE

The Greek philosopher Hippocrates, who is considered the Father of Medicine, emphasized in his regimen that if there is any deficiency in food or exercise, the body will fall sick.

Weight control and exercise go hand in hand. It is difficult to have one without the other. The body was made for movement. If you don't keep things moving, believe me, you won't be satisfied with what you see. If you let gravity take over, it will!

Balanced, nutrient dense meals combined with a suitable exercise program is perhaps the only way to keep excess weight off permanently.

You may painfully lose some weight, but probably not all you would like to by "dieting" alone. Calorie reduction slows the body's rate of metabolism and promotes fat storage.

Regular exercise actually increases the body's resting rate of metabolism and promotes fat burning. You not only burn off additional calories while performing the activity, you boost the rate at which you burn them all day long, even while you are doing nothing.

Couch Potato Syndrome

Speaking of doing nothing, did you know that your rate of metabolism actually slows down while you are watching television? The resting rate of metabolism is lower in someone watching television compared to the resting metabolism rate of someone sitting in a room doing absolutely nothing. If you read or perform some other activity such as needlework, your metabolism increases.

The benefits of exercise are so numerous they cannot possibly be all listed in a few pages so only a few major highlights will be pointed out.

1. Exercise promotes muscle tone (not bulk). Muscle cells burn fat for energy, so the more muscle you have, the easier it is to control fat.

NOTE: Some people are concerned that exercise promotes huge bulky muscles. Unless you genetically are prone to look this way anyway, strenuous training and a lot of calories are required daily. Body builders consume perhaps three to six times more calories than most people ever dream about, and many of them do use steriod hormones to further enhance muscular growth.

Exercising with light weights, walking, jogging, running, playing tennis, basketball, soccer, riding bike, swimming, hiking, roller blading, ice skating, etc., are for the most part aerobic exercises which help promote muscle tone and fat burning.

Remember: A pound of muscle takes up one-third the space as a pound of fat. When dieting, the results may be seen through the way your clothes fitter sooner than what the scale reflects.

2. Regular exercise increases your resting rate

of metabolism.

Muscles require oxygen to function. As we work them, their need for oxygen increases. The heart rates speeds up in order to carry oxygen to the muscles faster. As you continue to exercise and begin to tone your muscles, energy requirements increase.

3. Exercise promotes cardiovascular health by reducing LDL cholesterol and strengthening the heart and lungs.

4. Exercise lifts your spirits and relieves stress. You'll sleep better too!

NOTE: Exercise increases your need for protection against oxidation in the body and against tissue damage, so be sure to take lots of antioxidant nutrients such as Vitamin C (non-acidic), E, procyanidins, alpha lipoic acid, carotenes, zinc and chromium.

Antioxidants help prevent damage and shorten recovery time.

Getting the Most Out of Your Exercise Program

1. Exercise at the same time every day. Mornings are best because it boosts your resting metabolic rate for the entire day.

2. Get a training partner so you can encourage each other.

3. Listen to music or change your routine often to avoid boredom.

4. You need at least 12-20 minutes of aerobic exercise daily. You need to work hard enough so that your oxygen requirement increases so that your heart rate speeds up.

5. Other than a good pair of athletic shoes, you don't need any special equipment. You can jog in place, walk fast, do push ups, sit ups, calisthenics or jump rope.

6. Drink lots of water before, during and after your workout to avoid dehydration. Avoid sports drinks which are high in sugar and low in potassium.

7. If possible, get your body fat measured every two months. Remember, your progress cannot be monitored by what the scale says alone. Muscle takes up less space than fat so check the mirror and examine how your clothes fit.

TIPS FOR EVERYDAY LIVING

- Plan ahead. Try to prepare or plan your meals a day ahead of time. Avoid eating on the run. Impulsive food choices are more likely to be poor ones.

- Shop wisely. Don't shop for groceries when you're hungry – your impulses may override your good sense. Hit the outside aisles first. That's where the vegetables, fruits and grains, the basic foods you want to emphasize, are usually found.

- Cooking at home gives you more control over ingredients, cooking methods and cost. Home cooking doesn't have to be plain. Look at creating healthy, tasty meals as a challenge, not as a chore.

- If you are on the go a lot, you can easily carry fruit, bagels, even soup in a thermos and other healthy foods which can eliminate your need to stop somewhere and order something you should not. Plan ahead!

- Eat at least three small balanced meals every day. Do not skip meals, especially breakfast. Eating breakfast increases your resting metabolic rate for all day.

- Tighten your belt before meals.

- Drink a glass of water before you eat.

- Have a cup of clear soup and eat a salad (with low calorie dressing) 10-15 minutes before your meal.

• Eat more fiber. Fruits, vegetables, whole grains and beans add bulk and make one feel full.

• Eliminate sugar, cut down on simple carbohydrates and empty calories like sweets and alcohol. Avoid foods with a high glycemic index.

• Avoid all saturated fat. Avoid fried foods, fatty meats and skin from chicken.

• Eat slowly. Try to eat smaller bites and put your fork down in between bites.

• Chew your food well. Digestion begins in the mouth.

• Try putting meals on smaller plates.

• Use lemon juice, herbs and spices to flavor food instead of salt, butter, high calorie dressings and toppings.

• Don't worry about not losing weight fast enough. Your goal should be no more than one pound per week.

• Avoid commercial diets, liquid diets, etc., which can cause nutrient deficiencies and do not teach good eating habits.

• Don't allow dangerous snack foods in the home or workplace. Binging usually occurs at home so make these foods unavailable.

• If you are craving an "unhealthy" food, purchase the smallest amount possible to eliminate the possibility of emptying a large bag of it in one sitting or look for low-fat or a low-calorie version of the same food. For example, instead of ice cream, choose low-fat ice milk or frozen non-fat yogurt.

- Put on some of the clothes you would like to wear but are too tight.

- Fill up on water.

- Brush teeth and tongue.

- If you cannot resist the urge, eat low calorie fresh fruits or vegetables with a low glycemic value (cauliflower, broccoli, cucumbers, mushrooms, celery, apples, oranges, etc.).

- Avoid artificial sweeteners, for example, those found in diet drinks. Artificial sweeteners are many times sweeter than sugar so they cause a craving for sweets. In addition, artificial sweeteners may fool the body into thinking it has ingested sugar. As a result, your body releases extra insulin that can lead to weight gain.

- When you are offered a fattening food, remember that it probably provides no nutritional value what-so-ever and chose a better selection.

No-Guilt Snacks

Almost everybody likes to snack at least occasionally. **Fresh vegetables** are the best. They keep you busy, are crunchy and naturally low in calories. Keep a good supply of these on hand for this reason. Eat them whole and raw. Juicing eliminates valuable fiber that you need to make you feel full and carry fat out of the body.

Bibliography

Albanes, et al Alpha-tocopherol, Beta Carotene Cancer Protection Study Group. "The Effect of Vitamin E and Beta Carotene on the incidences of Lung Cancer and Other Cancer in Male Smokers." The New England H Journal of Medicine, Vol 330, 15 pg 1029-1035

Arai K; Miura J; Ohno M; Yokoyama J; Ikeda Y "Comparison of clinical usefulness of very-low-calorie diet and supplemental low-calorie diet." Am J Clin Nutr 1992 Jul;56(1 Suppl):275S-276S

Alger S; Larson K; et al "Effect of phenylpropanolamine on energy expenditure and weight loss in overweight women" National Institute of Diabetes and Digestive and Kidney Diseases, National Inst Am J Clin Nutr 1993 Feb;57(2):120-6

Anderson, Richard, "Exercise effects on chromium excretion of trained and untrained men consuming a constant diet" J Appl Physiol 64:249 (1988).

Airola, Paavo. *Hypoglycemia: A Better Approach* (1977) Health Plus Publishers, Phoenix, AZ.

American Heart Association *"The American Heart Association Diet* (1985) Dallas, TX.

Anderson, James, University of Kentucky, (Haysman and Hurley, The Healing Foods, Rodale Press, Emmaus, PA, (1989) pg 55.)

Atkins, Robert. *Dr. Atkins' Nutritional Breakthrough-How To Treat Your Medical Condition Without Drugs* (1979) Bantam Books, New York, NY.

Atkins, Robert and Shirley Linde. *Dr. Atkins' Super Energy Diet* (1977) Bantam Books, New York, NY.

Balch, James, Jr. M.D., and Phyllis, C.N.C., *Prescription for Nutritional Healing,* Avery Publishing, Garden City, N.Y. (1990).

Becker, E.W. et al "Clinical and biochemical evaluations of the alga spirulina with regards to its application in the treatment of obesity." Inst, Chem Pflanzenphysiologie. Nutrition Reports International, April 1986, Vol. 33, :4, 565.

Badmaev, V. ForsLean, **Ayurvedic Herb Coleaus forskohlii shows promise in enhancing lean body mass,** Health Supplement Retailer, July 2000. 30-32.

Bouchard C; Perusse L "Genetic aspects of obesity" Physical Activity Sciences Laboratory, Laval University, Ste-Foy, Quebec, Canada. *Ann N Y Acad Sci* (1993) Oct 29;699:26-35

Bulik CM "Abuse of drugs associated with eating disorders" J Subst Abuse 1992;4(1):69-90

Cheema-Dhadli S, Harlperin ML, Leznoff CC. Inhibition of enzymes which interact with citrate by (-)hydroxycitrate and 1,2,3,-tricarboxybenzene. Eur J Biochem 1973;38:98–102.

Chiang MT; Kimura S "Effect of dietary protein on the peroxidation of eicosapentaenoic acid in stroke-prone spontaneously hypertensive rats" Int J Vitam Nutr Res 1991;61(3):239-43

Chin C; Choy M "Cardiomyopathy induced by phenyl-propanolamine" J Pediatr 1993 Nov;123(5):825-7.

Cicalese L, Subbotin V, Rastellini C, et al. Acute rejection of small bowel allografts in rats: Protection afforded by pyruvate. Trans Proc 1996;28(5):2474.

Cicalese L, Lee K, Schraut W, et al. Pyruvate prevents ischemia-reperfusion mucosal injury of rat small intestine. Am J Surg 1996;171:97–101.

Cleary, M.P., Shepherd, P., Jenits, B., "Effect of dehydroepiandrosterone on growth in lean and obese Zucker rats." J Nutr, 1984; 114:1242-1251.

Clydesdale, FM "Carbohydrate Sweeteners in Nutrition; fact and fantasy." In Carbohydrates and Health, LF Hood and EK Wardip (eds.) pp. 128-132.

Coleman, D.L., Laiter, E.H.., Applerweig, N., "Therapeutic effects of dehydroepiandrosterone metabolities in diabetes mutant mice." Endocrinology, 1984; 115, 239-243.

Colgan, Michael, Ph.D., Optimum Sports Nutrition, Advanced Research Press, (1993) 202-203, 313-320.

Cunnane, S. "Preliminary Research on the Nutritional Effects of Flax in the Treatment of Cardiovascular Disease," Flax Research Priorities Conference, Flax Council of Canada, (March 1988).

Cynober, L. et al., Action of Ornithine alpha ketogluterate ornithine hydrochloride, and calcium alpha ketogluterate on plasma amino acids and hormonal patterns in healthy subjects. J American Coll Nutr 1990;9;2-12.

Davis BR; et al "Reduction in long-term antihypertensive medication requirements. Effects of weight reduction by dietary intervention in overweight persons with mild hypertension" Arch Intern Med 1993 Aug 9;153(15):1773-82

Deboer LWV, Bekx PA, Han L, et al. Pyruvate enhances recovery of rat hearts after ischemia and reperfusion by preventing free radical generation. Am J Physiol 1993;265:H1571–76.

Despres JP; Moorjani S; Lupien PJ; Tremblay A; Nadeau A; Bouchard C Genetic aspects of susceptibility to obesity and related dyslipidemias. Mol Cell Biochem 1992 Aug 18;113(2):151-69

Donnelly JE; Jakicic J; Gunderson S "Diet and body composition. Effect of very low calorie diets and exercise" Sports Med 1991 Oct;12(4):237-49

Donner MG; Schwandt P, Obesity stresses blood pressure and energy metabolism. What weight reduction really accomplishes] MMW Fortschr Med 1999 Dec 9;141(49-50):37-40.

Drazmin B., el al, eds, Insulin Action, New York Alan R. Liss, (1989)

Dudman NP; Wilcken DE; Stocker R Circulating lipid hydroperoxide levels in human hyperhomocysteinemia. Relevance to development of arteriosclerosis. Department of Cardiovascular Medicine, University of New South Wales, Prince Henry Hospital, Little Bay, Australia. Arterioscler Thromb 1993 Apr;13(4):512-6

Dunne, Lavon. Nutrition Almanac (1990) McGraw-Hill Publishing Company, New York, NY.

Elam, R.P., Morphological changes in adult men from resistance exercise and amino acid supplementation. J Sports Med. Phy Fit (1988) 28;35.

Eliasson K; et al "A dietary fibre supplement in the treatment of mild hypertension. A randomized, double-blind, placebo-controlled trial." J Hypertens 1992 Feb;10(2):195-9

Elliot DL, et al. Am J Clin Nutr 1989;49:93.

Erasmus, Udo. Fats and Oils (1986) Alive Books, Vancouver, British Columbia, Canada.

Ershler WB; Sun WH; Binkley N; et al.: Interleukin-6 and aging: blood levels and mononuclear cell production increase with advancing age and in vitro production is modifiable by dietary restriction. Lymphokine Cytokine Res 1993 Aug;12(4):225-30

Ensminger, A., et al, "Foods & Nutrition Encyclopedia, 2nd Edition," (1994) CRC Press, Boca Raton, FL

Enzi G, et al., eds. Obesity: Pathogenesis and Treatment. New York: Academic Press, 1981.

Evans, Gary, Ph.D, et al "A comparison of biological effects of chromium picolinate, chromium nicotinate and chromium chloride on skeletal muscle cells" J Inorganic Biochemistry (1992) 45.

Evans, Gary, Ph.D."An inexpensive, convenient conjunction for the treatment of diabetes" West J Med (1991) 155:549.

Evans, Gary, Ph.D.,"Cholesterol and glucose lowering effect of chromium picolinate." FASEB J (1989) 3:A761.

Evans, Gary, Ph.D. "Chromium picolinate: A review of clinical and animal studies" Lege Artis Medicine.

Evans, Gary, Ph.D., "Effects of Chromium picolinate on insulin controlled parameters in humans." Internat. J. Biosocial Med. Res 11(2):163-80 (1989)

Evian-Brion.D., et al, Simultaneous study of corticotropic pituitary secretions during ornithine infusion test, Clin Endocrinol 1982;17:119.

Feuers RJ; Weindruch R; Hart RW; "Caloric restriction, aging, and antioxidant enzymes" Mutat Res 1993 Dec;295(4-6):191-200

Felig P.; Clin Physiol (1984) 4:267-273

Fehlmann, M., Freycher P.; Biol Chem 256:7449 (1981)

Fischer, Jeffrey, M.D., "The Chromium Program" Harper and Row Publishers, New York (1990)

Fisher MC, La Chance PA.; Nutrition evaluation of published weight reducing diets. J Amer Dietet Assoc 1985;85:450-454.

Fisler JS; "Cardiac effects of starvation and semistarvation diets: safety and mechanisms of action." Am J Clin Nutr 1992 Jul;56(1 Suppl):230S-234S

Fukugawa, NK, Minaher KL, Rowe JW, et al.; J Clin Invest 76:2306 (1985)

Goran MI; Energy metabolism and obesity. Institute for Prevention Research, University of Southern California, Los Angeles,Med Clin North Am 2000 Mar;84(2):347-62.

Gordon, JB "An easy and inexpensive way to lower cholesterol?" West J Med (1991) 154:352.

Greenwood MRC, Cleary MP, Gruen R, et al.; Effect of (-)-hydroxycitrate on development of obesity in the Zucker obese rat. Am Phys J 1981;240:E72–78.

Hallmark, MA et al., "Effect of chromium supplementation and resistive training on muscle strength and lean body mass in untrained men" J Am Col Sports Med (1993)S101.

Hamilton, Eva May Nunnelley, Eleanor Noss Whitney, and Frances Sienkiewicz Sizer. Nutrition, Concepts and Controversies Third Edition (1979) West Publishing Company, St. Paul, MN.

Hasten, Deborah, et al; "Effects of Chromium picolinate on beginning weight training students" Int. J. Sports Nutrition 2:343-50 (1991) Health and Wellness Confidential (1988) Boardroom Reports, Inc, New York, NY.

Henrikson, R.: Earth Food Spirulina, Ronore Enterprises, Inc. Laguna Beach, Ca, (1989).

Hoffman, D.; The Herbal Handbook (1988) Healing Arts Press, Rochester, VT.

Howell, E.; Enzyme Nutrition, The Food Enzyme Concept (1985) Avery Publishing Group Inc., Wayne, NJ.

Isidori A. et al. A study of growth hormone release in man after oral administration of amino acids. Current Medical Research and Opinion 1981-7;475-481.

Ivy JL, Cortez MY, Chandler RM, et al. Effects of pyruvate on the metabolism and insulin resistance of obese Zucker rats. Am J Clin Nutr 1994;59:331–37.

Johnston, Ingeborg and James, "Flaxseed Oil and the Power of Omega-3" Keats Publishing, Inc., New Canaan, Conn, (1990).

Kamen, B. New Facts about Fiber, Nutrition Encounter, Novato, CA, 1991.

Kamrath RO; Plummer LJ; et al.; "Cholelithiasis in patients treated with a very-low-calorie diet." Am J Clin Nutr 1992 Jul;56(1 Suppl):255S-257S

Kaul L; Nidiry J "High-fiber diet in the treatment of obesity and hypercholesterolemia" *J Natl Med Assoc* 1993 Mar;85(3):231-2.

Kern PA, et al. The effect of weight loss on the activity and expression Qf adipose tissue lipoprotein lipase in very obese humans. N Engl J Med 1990;322: 1053.

Kimball, SR., Jefferson IS, Diabetes Metab Rev 4:773 (1988).

Kirkland L; Anderson R "Achieving healthy weights" Can Fam Physician 1993 Jan;39:157-8, 161-2.

Kaats, GR, Fisher JA, Blum K., "The effects of Chromium picolinate supplementation on body composition in different age groups" Age (1991)14:138.

Langer, Stephen. *Solved: The Riddle of Illness* (1984) Keats Publishing, Inc., New Canaan, CT.

Leung, Albert. *Chinese Herbal Remedies* (1984) Universe Books, New York, NY.

Lineback, David and George Inglett. *Food Carbohydrates* (1982) The AVI Publishing Company Inc., Westport, CT.

Lohman TG. Skinfolds and body density and their relation to body fatness: A review. Human Biol 1991;53:181-225.

Lowenstein JM. Effect of (-)-hydroxycitrate on fatty acid synthesis by rat liver in vivo. J Biol Chem 1971;246(3):629–32.

Malinow, M.R. et al. "Alfalfa" *American Journal of Clinical Nutrition,* (1979) 1,810-1,812.

McCarty, MF "Hypothesis: sensitization of insulin-dependent hypothalamic glucoreceptors may account for the fat-reducing effects of chromium picolinate" *J Optimal N* (1993) 2(1):36-53.

McCarty, MF "The case for supplemental chromium and a survey of clinical studies with chromium picolinate" *J Appl Nutr* (1991) 43:58-66

McCarty, MF "The prophylactic and therapeutic potential of chromium picolinate in diabetes, hyperlipidemia, anabolism and weight reduction" *J Adv. Med* (1993) 6:47-52.

Mensink, Ronald P. and Martijin B. Katan, "Effect of Dietary Trans-fatty Acids on High Density and Low Density Lipoprotein Cholesterol Levels in Healthy Subjects," *New England Journal of Medicine* (16 Aug 1990) *323 (7):* 439-445

Mindell, Earl. *Vitamin Bible* (1979) Warner Books, New York, NY.

Mindell, Earl. *Unsafe at Any Meal* (1987) Warner Books, Inc, New York, NY.

Molgaard, J., et al, "Alfalfa seeds lower low density lipoprotein B concentrations in patients with type II hyperlipoproteinemia" *Atherosclerosis* Vol 65 (1987) 173-179.

Morgan JP; Funderburk FR Phenylpropanolamine and blood pressure: a review of prospective studies. *Am J Clin Nutr* 1992 Jan;55(1 Suppl):206S-210S

Motulsky AG "Nutrition and genetic susceptibility to common diseases." *Am J Clin Nutr* 1992 Jun;55(6 Suppl):1244S-1245S

Nayaka, N. el al, "Cholesterol lowing effect of spirulina" Tokai University, Japan. *Nutrition Reports Int'l,* June 1988, Vol 37:6 132901337.

Nayaka, N. el al,"The effect of spirulina on reduction of serum cholesterol." TokaiUniv., Japan. *Progress in Medicine* Nov. 1986, Vol 6:11

Nestler, J.E., Clore, J.N., Blackard, W.G., "Metabolism and actions of dehydroepiandrosterone in humans." J Steroid Biochem Mol Biol, 1991; 40(6):599-605.

Nestler, J.E., Clore, J.N., Blackard, W.G., "Dehydroepiandrosterone: the missing link between hyperinsulinemia and atherosclerosis?: FASEB J, 1992 Sept; 6(12):3073-3075.

Netzer, Corinne, *The Complete Book Of Food Counts,* Dell Publishing, NY, New York (1991).

Oskai LB. The role of exercise in weight control. In: Wilmore JH, ed. Exercise and Sport Science Reviews Vol 1. New York: Academic Press, 1975:105-123.

Pac FA; Yigitoglu MR; Kalayci AG; Adam B; Atesal S; Kurkcuoglu M "Plasma lipid profile in obese children and in children with hereditary predisposition to coronary heart disease." *Jpn Heart J* 1992 Jul;33(4):445-50

Passwater, Richard, Ph.D., *Chromium Picolinate*, Keats Publishing (1992)

Pauling, Linus. *How to Live Longer and Feel Better* (1986) Avon Books, New York, NY.

Pauling, Linus. "Vitamin C and Common Cold and Flu" (1976) W.H. Freeman and Company, San Francisco, CA.

Pi-Sunyer FX"Short-term medical benefits and adverse effects of weight loss."Ann Intern Med 1993 Oct 1;119(7 Pt 2):722-6

Pittman CS, Suda AK, Chambers J, Jr, Ray GY, *Metabolism* 28:333 (1979)

Podell, Richard, M.D., *The G-Index Diet*, Warner Books, N.Y. New York (1993).

Press, RI, Geller, J., Evans GW.," The effect of chromium on serum and apolipoprotein fractions in human subjects." *West J Med* (1990)152-41-45.

Rasmussen MH; et al "Cimetidine suspension as adjuvant to energy restricted diet in treating obesity" *BMJ* 1993 Apr 24; 306(6885): 1093-6

Roehrig, Karla. *Carbohydrate Biochemistry and Metabolism* (1984) The AVI Publishing Company, Inc. Westport, CT.

Ravina A. Slezack L." The clinical use of the trace element chromium (III)in the treatment of diabetes mellitus. Harefuah

Reaven, G" Role of insulin resistance in human disease" *Diabetes,* 37:1595-1607,(1988).

Report of National Institute of Health Expert Panel on Weight-loss. Meeting at Bethesda, MD, 31 March - 2 April 1992.

Shoji T; Nishizawa Y; High-density-lipoprotein metabolism during a very-low-calorie diet Am J Clin Nutr 1992 Jul;56(1 Suppl):297S-298S

Seim HC; Holtmeier KB; "Effects of a six-week, low-fat diet on serum cholesterol, body weight, and body measurements." *Fam Pract Res J* 1992 Dec;12(4):411-9

Shannon, Ira L.; *Brand Name Guide to Sugar* (1977) Nelson-Hall Publishing, Chicago, ILL.

Simic MG; "The rate of DNA damage and aging" EXS 1992;62:20-30

Singh RB; Rastogi SS; Sircar AR; Mehta PJ; Sharma KK; "Dietary strategies for risk-factor modification to prevent cardiovascular diseases" *Nutrition* 1991 May-Jun;7(3):210-4

Spindler SR; Grizzle JM; Walford RL; Mote PL; "Aging and restriction of dietary calories increases insulin receptor mRNA, and aging increases glucocorticoid receptor mRNA in the liver of female C3B10RF1 mice." *J Gerontol* 1991 Nov;46(6):B233-7

Stanko RT, Mullick P, Clarke MR, et al.; Pyruvate inhibits growth of mammary adenocarcinoma 13762 in rats. Cancer Res1994;54:1004–1007.

Stanko RT, Reynolds HR, Hoyson R, et al. Pyruvate supplementation of a low-cholesterol, low-fat diet: Effects on plasma lipid concentration and body composition in hyperlipidemic patients. Am J Clin Nutr 1994;59:423–27.

Stanko RT, Robertson RJ, Galbreath RW, et al. Enhanced leg exercise endurance with a high-carbohydrate diet and dihyroxyacetone and pyruvate. J Appl Phys 1990;69(5):1651–56.

Stanko RT, Robertson RJ, Spina RJ, et al.; Enhancement of arm exercise endurance capacity with dihydroxyacetone and pyruvate. J Appl Phys 1990;68(1):119–24.

Stanko RT, Tietze DL, and Arch JE.; Body composition, energy utilization, and nitrogen metabolism with a 4.25-MJ/d low-energy diet supplemented with pyruvate. Am J Clin Nutr 1992;56(4):630–35.

Stone, Irwin.; *The Healing Factor: Vitamin C Against Disease* (1972) Putnam Publishing Group, New York, NY.

Sullivan AC, Hamilton JG, Miller ON, et al. Inhibition of lipogenesis in rat liver by (-)-hydroxycitrate. Arch Biochem Biophys 1972;150:183–90.

Sullivan AC, Triscari J. Metabolic regulation as a control for lipid disorders. Am J Clin Nutr 1977;30:767–76.

Sullivan AC, Triscari J, Hamilton JG, et al. Effect of (-)-hydroxycitrate upon the accumulation of lipid in the rat: I. Lipogenesis. Lipids 1974;9:121–128.

Sullivan AC, Triscari J, Hamilton JG, et al. Effect of (-)-hydroxycitrate upon the accumulation of lipid in the rat. II. Appetite. Lipids 1974;9(2):129–34.

Susser, Arnold. *The Indigestion of America From Headaches to Hemorrhoids* (1987) Nutrition Society of America, Westfield, NJ.

Treben, Maria. *Health Through God's Pharmacy* (1980) Wilhelm Ennsthaler, Steyr, Austria.

Triscari J, Sullivan AC; Comparative effects of (-)-hydroxycitrate and (=)-allo-hydroxycitrate on acetyl CoA carboxylase and fatty acid and cholesterol synthesis in vivo. Lipids 1977;12(4):357–63.

United States Environmental Protection Agency: "Preliminary Assessment of Suspected Carcinogens in Drinking Water" (1975) Report to Congress, Washington, D.C.

Valenzuela A; Morgado N; Trans fatty acid isomers in human health and in the food industry. Laboratorio de Lipidos y Antioxidantes, INTA, Universidad de Chile, Santiago, Chile. Biol Res 1999;32(4):273-87.

Van Gaal LF; Vansant GA; De Leeuw IH "Factors determining energy expenditure during very-low-calorie diets" Am J Clin Nutr 1992 Jul;56(1 Suppl):224S-229S

Vitale, Joseph, and Selwyn Broitman. *Advances in Human Clinical Nutrition* (1982) John Wright PSG Inc. Boston, MA.

Wade, Carlson. *Amino Acids Book* (1985) Keat's Publishing, Inc. New Canaan, CT.

Walford RL; Harris SB; Gunion MW "The calorically restricted low-fat nutrient-dense diet in Biosphere 2 significantly lowers blood glucose, total leukocyte count, cholesterol, and blood pressure in humans." Proc Natl Acad Sci U S A 1992 Dec 1;89(23):11533-7

Wang BY; et al; "Dietary arginine prevents atherogenesis in the coronary artery of the hypercholesterolemic rabbit." Division of Cardiovascular Medicine, Stanford University School of Medicine, J Am Coll Cardiol 1994 Feb;23(2):452-8

Wang GJ; Volkow ND; Logan J; Pappas NR; Wong CT; Zhu W; Netusil N; Fowler JS
Brain dopamine and obesity. Department of Medicine, Brookhaven National Laboratory, Upton, New York Lancet 2001 Feb 3;357(9253):354-7.

Webster, James. *Vitamin C: The Protective Vitamin* (1972) Universal-Award House, Inc., New York, NY.

Weil, Andrew. Natural Health, *Natural Medicine* (1990) Houghton Mifflin Company, Boston, MA.

Weindruch R, "Effect of caloric restriction on age-associated cancers" Exp Gerontol 1992 Sep-Dec;27(5-6):575-81

Index

ORDER THESE GREAT BOOKS
FROM BL PUBLICATIONS!

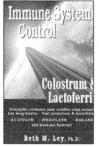

Immune System Control
Colostrum & Lactoferrin
Beth M. Ley, Ph.D. 200 pages, $12.95 ISBN 1-890766-11-9
Get the indepth and detailed FACTS about colostrum and lactoferrin! Testimonials and much more! Also features a special product selection guide! Fully referenced/Indexed

Marvelous Memory Boosters
Beth M. Ley, Ph.D. 2000, 32 pages, $3.95

Certain nutrients & phytochemicals (Alpha GPC, Vinpocetine, Huperzine-A, Pregnenolone, Phospholipids, DHA, Bacopa Monniera, Ginkgo Biloba, etc.) improve short & long term memory, increase mental acuity & concentration, improve learning abilities & mental stamina, reduce fatigue, improve sleep, mood, vision & hearing.

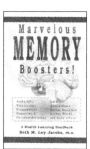

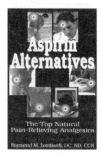

Aspirin Alternatives:
The Top Natural Pain-Relieving Analgesics
Raymond Lombardi, D.C., N.D., C.C.N., 1999, 160 pages, $8.95

This book discusses analgesics and natural approaches to pain. Ibuprofen and acetaminophen are used for pain-relief, but like all drugs, there is a risk of side effects and interactions, There are a number of natural alternatives which are equally effective and in many cases may be preferable because they may help treat the underlining problem rather than simply treating a symptom.

Vinpocetine: Boost Your Brain w/ Periwinkle
Extract! Beth M. Ley, Ph.D. 2000, 48 pgs. $4.95

This herbal extract benefits: Memory, attention and concentration, learning, circulation, hearing, insomnia, depression, tinnitus, vision & more! Vinpocetine increases circulation in the brain and increases metabolism in the brain by increasing use of glucose and oxygen. Benefits both the old and young!

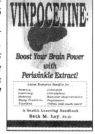

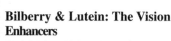

Bilberry & Lutein: The Vision
Enhancers
Beth M. Ley, Ph.D. 40 pgs. $4.95

Find out how bilberry and lutein, important antioxidants specifically for the eyes, can help improve your vision and ward off common eye problems including macular degeneration, cataracts, glaucoma, retinopathy, etc.

118

**God Wants You Well: How to Obtain Freedom
from Illness and Disease** Beth M. Ley, Ph.D. 2001
260 pages, $14.95

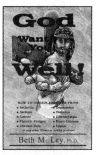

*Find out which foods can not only help you prevent com-
mon health problems such as diabetes, cancer and heart
disease, but which foods to avoid. Find out what God
wants from you so you can be free of health problems. The
Bible gives us awesome insight on how we are to take care
of our bodies and what we need to be whole.*

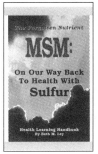

**MSM: On Our Way Back To Health With
Sulfur** Beth M. Ley, 1998, 40 pages, $3.95

*MSM (methyl sulfonyl methane), is a rich source of
organic sulfur, important for connective tissue regenera-
tion. Beneficial for arthritis and other joint problems,
allergies, asthma, skin problems, TMJ, periodontal conditions, pain relief, and much more!
Includes important "How to use"
directions.*

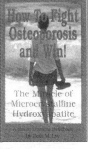

**How to Fight Osteoporosis & Win: The Miracle
of MCHC** Beth M. Ley, 80 pgs. $6.95

*Find out if you are at risk for osteroporosis and what to do
to prevent and reverse it. Get the truth about bone loss,
calcium, supplements, foods, MCHC & much more! Find
out what supplements can help you most!*

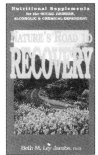

Nature's Road to Recovery: Nutritional
**Supplements for The Social Drinker, Alcoholic &
Chemical-Dependent**
Beth M. Ley-Jacobs, Ph.D., 1999, 72 pages, $5.95

*Recovery involves much more than abstinence. Cravings,
depression, memory loss, liver problems, vascular problems, sexual problems, sleep problems, nutritional deficiencies and common health problems which can benefit
from 5-HTP, DHA, phospholipids, St.
John's Wort, antioxidants, etc.*

DHA: The Magnificent Marine Oil
Beth M. Ley-Jacobs, Ph.D., 1999, 120 pages, $6.95

*Individuals commonly lack this essential Omega-3 fatty
acid so important to the brain, vision, and immune system
and much more. Memory, depression, ADD, addiction disorders (especially alcoholism), inflammatory disorders,
skin problems, schizophrenia, elevated blood lipids, etc.,
benefit from DHA.*

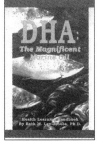

T O   P L A C E   A N   O R D E R :

___ *Aspirin Alternatives: The Top Natural Pain-Relieving Analgesics* (Lombardi) $8.95

___ *Discover the Beta Glucan Secret!* (Ley) $3.95

___ *Bilberry & Lutein: The Vision Enhancers!* (Ley) $4.95

___ *Calcium: Fossilized Coral* (Ley) $4.95

___ *Castor Oil: Its Healing Properties* (Ley) $3.95

___ *Dr. John Willard on Catalyst Altered Water* (Ley) $3.95

___ *Co Q10: All-Around Nutrient for All-Around Health* (Ley) . $4.95

___ *Colostrum: Nature's Gift to the Immune System* (Ley) $5.95

___ *DHA: The Magnificent Marine Oil* (Ley Jacobs) $6.95

___ *DHEA: Unlocking the Secrets of the Fountain of Youth - 2nd Edition* (Ash-Ley) $14.95

___ *Fading: One family's journey with a women silenced by Alzheimer's* (Kraft) $12.95

___ *God Wants You Well* (Ley) $14.95

___ *Health Benefits of Probiotics* (Dash) $4.95

___ *How to Fight Osteoporosis and Win!* (Ley) $6.95

___ *How Did We Get So Fat? 2nd Edition* (Susser/Ley) $8.95

___ *Immune System Control-Colostrum & Lactoferrin* (Ley) $12.95

___ *Marvelous Memory Boosters* (Ley) $3.95

___ *Medicinal Mushrooms:* **Agaricus blazei Murill** *(Ley)* . .$4.95

___ *MSM: On Our Way Back to Health W/ Sulfur* (Ley) $3.95

___ *Natural Healing Handbook* (Ley) $14.95

___ *Nature's Road to Recovery: Nutritional Supplements for the Alcoholic & Chemical Dependent* (Ley Jacobs) $5.95

___ *PhytoNutrients: Medicinal Nutrients Found in Foods* (Ley) . $3.95

___ *The Potato Antioxidant: Alpha Lipoic Acid* (Ley) $6.95

___ *Vinpocetine: Revitalize Your Brain w/ Periwinkle Extract!* (Ley) $4.95

___ *Yesterday, Today & Tomorrow: Take the High Road to Health with Rod Burreson* (Burreson) $24.95

Book subtotal $ _____   Please add $4.00 for shipping

TOTAL $_____

Send check or money order to:
BL Publications 14325 Barnes Drive Detroit Lakes, MN 56501

Credit card orders call toll free: 1-877-BOOKS11
visit: www.blpbooks.com